Self Care

Reiki Guide to Enhance Psychic Abilities and Mindpower Using Guided Meditation

(Achieve a Higher Level of Consciousness and Spiritual Energy)

Penelope Ewing

Published by Rob Miles

Penelope Ewing

All Rights Reserved

Self Care: Reiki Guide to Enhance Psychic Abilities and Mindpower Using Guided Meditation (Achieve a Higher Level of Consciousness and Spiritual Energy)

ISBN 978-1-989990-37-7

All rights reserved. No part of this guide may be reproduced in any form without permission in writing from the publisher except in the case of brief quotations embodied in critical articles or reviews.

Legal & Disclaimer

The information contained in this book is not designed to replace or take the place of any form of medicine or professional medical advice. The information in this book has been provided for educational and entertainment purposes only.

The information contained in this book has been compiled from sources deemed reliable, and it is accurate to the best of the Author's knowledge; however, the Author cannot guarantee its accuracy and validity and cannot be held liable for any errors or omissions. Changes are periodically made to this book. You must consult your doctor or get professional medical advice before using any of the suggested remedies, techniques, or information in this book.

Upon using the information contained in this book, you agree to hold harmless the Author from and against any damages, costs, and expenses, including any legal fees potentially resulting from the application of any of the information provided by this guide. This disclaimer applies to any damages or injury caused by the use and application, whether directly or indirectly, of any advice or information presented, whether for breach of contract, tort, negligence, personal injury, criminal intent, or under any other cause of action.

You agree to accept all risks of using the information presented inside this book. You need to consult a professional medical practitioner in order to ensure you are both able and healthy enough to participate in this program.

TABLE OF CONTENTS

INTRODUCTION 1

CHAPTER 1: LEARNING REIKI 3

CHAPTER 2: THE THREE DEGREES 19

CHAPTER 3: HISTORY OF REIKI... 36

CHAPTER 4: REIKI: AN INTRODUCTION 47

CHAPTER 5: CLEARING YOUR ENERGY FIELD.................... 60

CHAPTER 6: PRINCIPLES OF REIKI 66

CHAPTER 7: CLEANSING YOUR ENERGY 69

CHAPTER 8: REIKI TREATMENT 77

CHAPTER 9: REIKI LIFESTYLE 87

CHAPTER 10: LIFE WITH THREE EYES.............................. 105

CHAPTER 11: HISTORY OF REIKI...................................... 115

CHAPTER 12: THE REIKI HEALING TECHNIQUES 123

CHAPTER 13: INTRODUCTION TO THE GUIDED MEDITATIONS 129

CHAPTER 14: THE EASTERN VERSION 136

CHAPTER 15: MEDITATION AND REIKI 150

CHAPTER 16: AN OVERVIEW... 155

CHAPTER 17: REIKI: IN-DEPTH EXPLANATION 161

CHAPTER 18: HOW IS HEALING EXPECTED TO BE OBTAINED FROM USING THIS MEDICATION TECHNIQUES 166

CHAPTER 19: USING REIKI ON YOURSELF 175

CHAPTER 20: THE ORIGIN AND HISTORY OF REIKI 189

CHAPTER 21: ORIGINS AND HISTORY OF REIKI 199

CONCLUSION 202

Introduction

Reiki is basically pronounced as "Ray-Key" which is derived from a Japanese word means universal energy. The work Reiki has been heard a lot of times but less people know about it. It has been a practice in many of the countries since a long time and now getting popular since people have started to feel the symptoms even more now. The symptoms such as stress, anxiety, depression, anger and much more has rose in people due to the busy lives.

They are not able to focus on their life due to which they have been exposed to the negative energies attacking them. Reiki works as a well-being for the human beings. It is just the flowing of hands which are done on your head, hands, feet and external parts which are visible from your clothes to make you feel better. You do not take off your clothes for the massage but the main parts get a massage by releasing the tension from your body.

If you are someone who has not no exposure of Reiki then make sure to get it done once in a lifetime. It is session where you do not have to do anything but the practitioner does all for you. The environment of reiki is pleasant by making you feel comfortable. It is basically 15 minutes session which you can attend and make the best out of your life. You will feel a change in your mood with feeling lighter and easier on life. You will take things positively and will work as a conflict resolution for your life.

Chapter 1: Learning Reiki

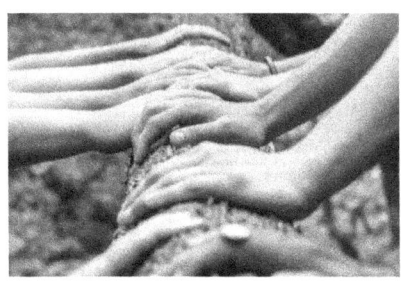

Reiki energy healing is a traditional Japanese healing style. It involves the flow of universal energy as it is channeled through a Reiki practitioner. Reiki is performed with a series of static hand positions that can be placed directly on the body for direct contact or performed hands off, with the hands hovering above the body.

Translated, Reiki is broken into two words. Rei translates into 'Universe' and Ki translates into 'Energy' the same as Qi, or Chi. Reiki means Universal Energy.

The universe is made up of energy. Everything in the universe is made up of energy. Reiki practitioners can connect to that energy on a profound level. Channeling the energy through themselves it can then be used to heal and balance other energetic currents, like the ones found in the human body.

The man most credited for the discovery of Reiki is Dr. Mikao Usui. Dr. Usui grew up in Japan in a family that followed Zen Buddhism traditions. He was born in 1865. After Dr. Usui fell ill during a cholera epidemic, he had a spiritual awakening while he was fighting for his life.

Upon recovering, Dr. Usui went to a Zen monastery where he began his spiritual studies. During his studies, he came across Reiki, a method of healing that had been used for centuries. This healing method used a set of hand positions and symbols that amplified and channeled the energy for healing.

Dr. Usui wanted to use Reiki to heal others, but he felt like he needed more awareness before implementing the healing process. For this awakening he looked inward and started to meditate and practice meditation.

According to legend, as a part of his spiritual journey, he traveled up Mt. Kurama. When he was on the mountain top, he gathered twenty-stones and then he sat down to meditate. For each day that passed on this meditation, Dr. Usui would throw away one of the stones he had gathered. He spent his entire time meditating and studying.

After twenty-one days had passed, Usui opened himself up with the intention of wanting to see things clearly. It was during this time that it is said a bright light flashed above him and rushed towards him. The light beamed through his forehead and Usui saw the Reiki symbols that he had been studying in Sutras at the Zen monastery. It is thought that in this moment, he experienced spiritual enlightenment.

On his travel back down the mountain, legend tells that Usui hurt his foot, and he instinctively placed his hand over his foot, observing that the bleeding stopped and the pain diminished.

Later, Dr. Usui stopped in a village and was given a full meal. He was able to eat the complete meal without any discomfort, despite having been fasting and meditating for twenty-one days. The girl who gave him his meal was experiencing pain and he was able to heal her as well. Upon returning to the monastery, Usui used his healing gift to heal his superior who was suffering from arthritis pain.

Dr. Usui set out on the noble venture of using Reiki to heal the homeless and poor people of Kyoto. He used Reiki in hopes of helping beggars become more productive member of society. Unfortunately, he became discouraged when he found them returning to their habits or begging.

Through this experience, Usui was reminded that it is essential to heal the body, mind, and soul for there to be change. He retreated into meditation again. During this meditation, Usui discovered the five principles of Reiki. He spent the remainder of his life practicing and teaching Reiki.

In April of 1922, Usui established a Reiki center where he taught Reiki to students and performed sessions for the public.

Traditional Reiki is broken into three levels or degrees of Reiki. The first degree of Reiki is called Shoden (First Degree) and was divided into four levels: Loku-Tou, Go-Tou, Yon-Tou, and San-Tou. The second degree of Reiki is known as Okuden (Inner Teaching) and has two levels: Okuden-Zen-ki (first part) and Okuden-Koe-ki (Second part). The third degree of Reiki is called Shinpiden (Mystery Teaching) and is now called the Master Level.

Chujiro Hayashi was a retired marine and a physician before he began studying Reiki with Usui. As a request from Usui before he died, Hayashi opened his own Reiki clinic to spread the teachings and expand the development of Reiki.

Hayashi kept very meticulous, careful records of the people he treated at his clinic. He kept records of illnesses and conditions and made notes on which Reiki positions and symbols had the best results with various conditions. With his notes and observations, Hayashi wrote Reiki Ryoho Shinshin, which means Guidelines for Reiki Healing Method. He used this guide as a manual in his classes.

In his clinic, Hayashi changed the way Reiki sessions were given and received. He didn't just have clients sit in a chair, but he had them lie on a treatment table. He also began the practice of group sessions where one client would receive simultaneous treatments from several practitioners at once. He developed a new system for giving Reiki Attunements as well.

Hayashi began to change the way Reiki was taught. When he traveled, he would teach the Shoden and Okuden (Reiki degree I and II) together in one seminar that spanned five days. Each day included two or three hours of class instruction as well as one attunement.

Prior to the attack on Pearl Harbor, Hayashi traveled to Hawaii. The Japanese military asked him to report any information on warehouses and military targets in Honolulu. Hayashi refused to make such reports and was thus labeled a traitor by the Japanese government. In 1940, Hayashi performed seppuku (ritual suicide) in order to restore his families honor.

Hawayo Takata is the Reiki Master how is most credited with bringing Reiki to the western world. She also is credited with the growth, development, and expansion of modern Reiki, Reiki teachings, and the spread of Reiki influence.

Takata was born in Hawaii in 1900. Her parents were Japanese immigrants. Takata married a bookkeeper or the plantation where she was also employed. They had two daughters. When her husband died in 1930, Takata had to take on all the labor of her family.

After five years, she began to develop severe abdominal pain and a lung condition. This led to a nervous breakdown. Soon after her breakdown, one of Takata's sisters died and she had to travel to Japan in order to inform her parents who had moved back to their native country.

Takata went into a hospital in Japan for her abdominal pain and the lung condition. She was diagnosed with a tumor and gallstones, asthma, and appendicitis. Rather than getting surgery, Takata went to visit Hayashi's clinic.

Never having experienced Reiki before, Takata was curious, and she was impressed that the diagnosis from the Reiki practitioner was very close to the one she received in the hospital. It was then that Takata began receiving Reiki treatments.

She wanted to learn how to perform Reiki and began to work in Hayashi's clinic and study Reiki. After working in the clinic for a year, she reached her Shinpiden Attunement, Master level.

Takata returned to Hawaii and she began to practice Reiki, opening several clinics. She gave treatments and would teach students up to level II Reiki. She traveled throughout the US and the world, becoming a renowned healer.

After 1970, Takata began teaching students and attuning them to the Master Level, but for a fee of $10,000 for a weekend of training. Usui did not have a high fee for his teachings, and it is speculated that Takata charged a high fee to create respect and credibility for the Reiki discipline.

Takata did not believe that treatments and teachings should be given for free. She did not provide her students with written course material and forbade them from taking notes or recordings. When she taught the Reiki symbols, she made her students memorize them and did not allow them to draw them out or make copies of them.

Traditionally, Reiki was taught orally, and Takata wanted to keep that the traditional teaching method. Although neither Usui or Hayashi stuck to oral traditions. Takata received a Reiki manual from Hayashi during her studies.

Takata changed the way that Reiki was taught by simplifying and refining the hand positions she had been taught.

By the time Takata died in 1980, she had attuned and initiated twenty-two Reiki masters. She made her students promise to keep teaching Reiki the same way that she had taught them.

This teaching avenue made Reiki a rather exclusive organization in both Japan and the US. Over time though, Masters that Takata had trained began to lower their fees. This changed the way Reiki was taught with more of an emphasis on the wisdom of Reiki guiding the sessions.

Reiki classes became more open and accessible. Using workbooks and printed study material came back into practice. Students were encouraged to study under different practitioners and Masters for a more well-rounded learning experience. These shifts allowed for Reiki to become more widely taught. It is estimated that there are now over four million Reiki practitioners in the world and over one million Reiki Masters.

When learning and studying Reiki there are going to be several methods for your learning experience. Some Masters will teach more traditionally, breaking the course up into the three degrees, teaching each level individually. Each level might be a weekend long class experience with additional work to perform on your own before progressing to the next level.

Some Masters might condense all three degrees into one weekend long seminar and then encourage you to continue studying and working on your own to hone your skills. With the spread of technology and online courses that are readily available, some Masters have brought their teachings to online courses.

Sometimes online courses are more practical because you can work at your own pace and don't need to stick to a strict schedule. This means you can work around your own busy lifestyle and still learn. You won't have to take time off or even travel to a Master for a weekend course. Since Reiki can be performed over distances, then doing online course work and then getting your Attunements from a distance, is just as effective.

Some Reiki courses do provide their students with excellent course material for study. Some courses might require students to do continued work outside of the class. A common follow up practice to Reiki Level I could be to perform twenty-one self-healing Reiki session on consecutive days. This is to simulate Usui's twenty-one days of meditation.

After receiving your Reiki Level II attunement, you might be required to perform five consecutive self-treatments, five consecutive treatments on someone else, and five consecutive distance treatments. These treatments should incorporate the Reiki symbols when possible.

Whether you decide to take an online course or study Reiki in an in-person seminar or class setting, make sure to accurately and seriously complete any assignments that are given to you. In order to get the most out of your study, you are going to want to treat it like any other class. If an assignment is to draw out the Reiki symbols on a piece of paper every day for a week, that may seem silly and time consuming, but cutting corners in the coursework won't give you the best learning experience.

Regardless of if you are taking an online course or an in-person course, you should find a Reiki Master that you can talk to, share experiences with, and get sessions from. Maybe they'll even trade sessions with you. This Reiki Master doesn't necessarily have to be the Master that you are learning from in your courses. Having a mentor of sorts will greatly enhance your experience in learning Reiki.

When deciding what kind of course to take, do your research on the Master that is teaching the course. What is their experience level? Do they have good reviews? Do their students have success in their field after the course? Does the course have any kind of standardized testing or take-home work?

You'll want to look for courses that meet your own needs, but you'll also want to find a course that is going to be worth your time and money. Don't be discouraged or turned off to a course just because it is online. Don't think that a course lacks credibility because it teaches Reiki Level I and II in one seminar.

There are so many ways to learn Reiki now. This is both a blessing and a possible curse. You should easily be able to find a course style that fits with your schedule and life. However, since it is so easy for Masters to post a generic online course that they just post PowerPoint presentations for, you'll want to be careful not to get into a course that doesn't have to merit or information that you are seeking.

Usui Reiki is also called Traditional Reiki. This is the Reiki discipline that has the three degrees of Reiki. There are other Reiki traditions that have developed that can have nine degrees to learn. This book is primarily going to cover information that is aligned with Traditional Reiki.

When studying Reiki, it is important to remember that you don't need to learn beyond Reiki Level I if you do not feel called to. Reiki Level II and the Master

Level do provide additional tools for Reiki, deepen your connection to Reiki energy, and also offer advanced Reiki Techniques. However, if you are comfortable with Reiki Level I, there may not be a need to progress.

Reiki Attunements last forever, so you only need to receive the Attunements once. Reiki is a skill though and does require practice to keep those skills sharp. There are some cases in which a Reiki Master may ask you to receive additional Attunements. If you took Reiki Level I and then sought a different Master for Reiki Level II, they might require you to receive both Reiki Level I and II attunements from them.

If you studied Reiki eleven years ago and then decided to get back into it, your Master might require you to get the Attunements again if you take a refresher course. While you won't need the Attunements to practice Reiki, it doesn't hurt to get them and help reopen those channels, especially if you haven't actively been practicing Reiki.

You can use Reiki as a self-healing method only, or as a professional healing service to heal paying clients. If you do decide to see clients, it is recommended that you at least progress through Reiki Level II. This isn't required and many Reiki Level I practitioners have successful businesses. Reiki Level II will simply increase your knowledge of Reiki, attune you to the Reiki Symbols, and deepen your wisdom. This can create a more powerful healing experience for yourself and others.

There is no harm in taking a Reiki level I course and then staying at that level until you feel called to progress to the next level. You may never feel called to. It might take months, or years for you to feel like you want to move forward with your studies. Wherever you are comfortable in your spiritual journey is where you should be.

Chapter 2: The Three Degrees

The father of modern Reiki, Mikao Usui, was born on August 15th, 1865, in what is known today as the town of Taniai-Mura located in the Yamagata area of Gifu in the modern-day prefecture of Kyoto. Not much is known about Mikao Usui, but it is believed that he was born within a wealthy family as only the male children of wealthy families were able to have access to above average education.

From an early age, Usui trained within the Buddhist religion at the Tendai Buddhist school. He began schooling within this discipline as a very young child. He quickly began training in disciplined of ever-increasing difficulty. He is recalled as a gifted child who showed promise in a number of areas such as prescription, fortune telling, studies of the brain and the mind, and deep religious philosophy. As a result of his studies, he was able to take advantage of every opportunity to learn the ways of the world and the way the human body and mind functioned together. His understanding of the Buddhist Bible, the Kyoten, was very deep and insightful. He eventually married to a young lady named Sadako. The couple had a girl born around 1907.

As an adult, Usui had deep curiosity about the ways of the world outside of his home country. He ventured out into China and some western countries. In doing so, he was able to learn about the ways in which people conducted themselves in cultures different to his. Usui held a number of different positions such as office worker, neighborhood officer, a reporter, secretary to a legislator, chairman to convicts and even an industrialist. He would serve as secretary to Shimpei Goto, who was a renowned government official in the position of Secretary of the Railroad, then later serving the Postmaster General and ultimately becoming Secretary of the Interior and the State.

Nevertheless, Usui ended up foregoing this lifestyle and took up the habits of the Buddhist Monks. He would eventually enter the Buddhist priesthood thus cementing his life's purpose. He would consistently reflect on the meaning of life while undergoing the 21 days of suffering. It is said that during these sufferings, Usui received a divine inspiration for a plan of physical recovery which would eventually be known as "Reiki". This story is said to have happened on Mount Kurama during one of his sufferings.

The overall inspiration is believed to have been a combination of a series of traditional oriental treatments, fused into one, and harmonized to create a holistic approach to healing the body. As such, Reiki shares its origins with traditional Chinese medicine, the oriental discipline Chi Gong and the Japanese Kiko needle treatment. By experimenting with the techniques of all these disciplines, Usui discovered the extraordinary results on a number of ailments.

By April 1922, Usui began teaching this healing art at the first school of its kind in Harajuku, Tokyo. At first, Usui had a small handbook which was later translated into

English and disseminated in the Western world. The handbook's original title was "The Original Reiki Handbook of Dr. Mikao Usui" as published by the early Reiki master Frank Arjava Petter, who was living in Japan at the time.

Due to Usui's track record of success, his fame as a doctor and healer began spreading across Japan. Given the fact that Japan was undergoing a deep and profound social change, this apparent revolution coincided with Japan's aperture to the West.

Reiki thus began gaining a foothold among people of all sorts, but in particular, Reiki quickly gained momentum with older individuals who believed in preserving their ties to ancient healing practices.

At the first Reiki school, learners were taught Reiki as a means of healing, but also as a way of preserving Japan's cultural legacy and history. History records that this school gained notoriety as the number of learners that attended it began to increase.

In September of 1923, a massive earthquake rocked Tokyo and Yokohoma. It is believed that this earthquake measure 7.9 on the Richter Scale. It left thousands of dead and even more wounded. It is believed that the number of casualties from this earthquake was around 140,000. At its time, it was the single-most destructive event in Japanese history. But it also afforded Usui, and his students, the opportunity to put their Reiki discipline to the test. They would go out to treat those who had been injured in the earthquake. As a result of this effort, Reiki began to garner a great deal of attention.

By 1925, Usui's following had grown to the degree that he was looking to open a second school in Nakano, located outside of Tokyo. As Usui began to spend time away from the first school, his senior students began taking over his duties. These senior students began training other novice learners in the ways of Reiki. However, Usui passed away before he could complete the opening of the second school. His death in 1926 spurred the construction of a monument in his honor near his grave at the Saihoji Temple y Suginamiku, Tokyo. His followers would honor Usui's legacy by continuing to teach Reiki.

Reiki would eventually be divided into 6 different levels of mastery. The first four are known as "Shoden" with the last two are known as "Okuden" in addition to the Shinpi-nook. In the beginning levels, disciplines are asked to master their presence and relationship with the material (Shoden) before progressing into the deeper, inward levels (Okuden). After these levels, the disciple arrives at the Shinpi-lair level, or the mystery level. Under this construction, around 2,000 individuals were trained in the ways of Reiki with a total of about 15 to 17 Reiki masters. Although, it should be noted that there was no such title of "Reiki Master" at the time in Japan.

Reiki is known to be a difficult discipline to master. There are three tiers before students arrive at mastery of Reiki. Nevertheless, time and effort are needed before arriving at full mastery of each level. Here is a description of the three tiers or degrees.

The first degree, known as Reiki, I or Shoden is the introductory phrase in which students learn about history and the underlying philosophy of Reiki. Also, students are taught how to offer Reiki to others and channel the healing energy to the ailing individual.

The second degree, known as Reiki II, or Okuden, students are introduced to the "secret" ways of Reiki. The student is then asked to deepen their learning of the healing energy offered through Reiki. At the completion of this degree, the student is regarded as a "Reiki Master".

The third degree, known as Reiki III, or Shinpinden, is when the master attains the level needed to become a teacher of Reiki. In this degree, training is often split up into parts, one is the attunement of the healing energy while the second part is devoted to honing the master's teaching ability.

Now, let's take a deeper look into the each of the Reiki degrees.

First Degree Of Reiki: Shoden Self Treatment

Shoden is a Japanese word signifying "first lessons".

It is the main degree of lessons in the customary Japanese part of Reiki called Usui Reiki Ryoho.

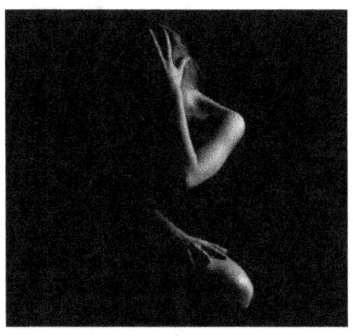

Vitality is a word that not many individuals can clarify in the entirety of its complexities. You could peruse a book on it or be informed all concerning it however it is simply the genuine encounter that educates you.

In this way, a total treatment is given and gotten by each taking an interest understudy and numerous hands-on activities are utilized in a gathering situation during Shoden. This useful experience prompts an internal comprehension of vitality.

A great part of the course is spent working from this perspective, instructing you to work instinctively and to bring that instinctual balance into your regular day-to-day existence. For a fact, it takes, in any event, two days to pick up this degree of certainty. The strategies used to encourage this depend on both the experiential information, which you gain all through the course just as your very own understanding of specialized capacity.

Conventional Japanese Reiki reflection strategies are educated and rehearsed over the two days to expand on this lively information and to help your mending procedure.

In the wake of finishing Shoden in-person, the understudy is approached to keep rehearsing on oneself and complete the online lessons at the Ki Campus. This proceeds with the lively clearing, which was started during the course itself.

Mending resembles 'making entire'; making a balance in your life. The International House of Reiki sees the contemplating of the arrangement of Reiki as an otherworldly venture – one that is embraced by you with each help offered during, and after, the course by the educators.

Advantages of Shoden Reiki:

Figure out how to unwind.

Increase an unmistakable comprehension of vitality work.

Experience enthusiastic and physical discharge.

Feel good with yourself.

Build up your caring and cherishing perspectives.

Help other people.

Feel solid.

Be educated about the arrangement of Reiki.

Get individual continuous consideration and direction from your instructor.

Have a place with a universal mending network, the International House of Reiki, and get every one of the advantages of the middle's incredible emotionally supportive networks. Shoden understudies are urged to resist for a base charge for proceeding with instruction purposes.

Second Degree of Reiki: Okuden Self Treatment

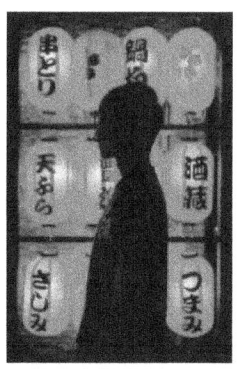

The Second Degree (Okuden) Reiki; instructs understudies to grasp instinctive working, increasing trust in removed, non-contact Reiki with the utilization of hallowed vitality images to reinforce your association and help you on your adventure. This is anything but essential expertise for the vast majority to have, and it is more inside and out than the clear First-Degree Reiki.

Experiencing Okuden preparing is prescribed for understudies who have taken Shoden level 1 course and have been rehearsing day by day self-treatment for at least a half year. The Reiki Intuitive recommends understudies who have prepared with another Master to either have a discussion or go to her Reiki Share bunch before focusing on the preparation in full.

Okuden is a Japanese word signifying 'inward lessons'. As the word suggests a more profound comprehension and association with Usui Mikao's lessons is accomplished during this course.

This level instructs how to associate with Earth and Heaven vitality, the initial steps to winding up completely incorporated with the universe. This is accomplished through the act of Shirushi (images) and

Jumon (mantras). It will empower the understudy to upgrade his/her very own vitality levels and affectability. There are numerous viewpoints to the Shirushi and Jumon which incorporate reciting and perception strategies. As opposed to being outside apparatuses – the attention here is on inner use for otherworldly improvement.

The idea of Oneness, understanding that we are One vigorously with everything known to mankind, is one of the significant advantages of working as such and is normally drilled in the course. A component of this investigation of Oneness enables the professional to see the more profound implications of far off mending. Extra Japanese Reiki strategies are offered to help profound development significantly further.

As mindfulness develops so does the capacity to help other people – this is talked about at this level. In the wake of finishing Okuden, the understudy is required to proceed with the rehearsing on oneself as well as other people where conceivable.

Advantages of Okuden Reiki:

Discover balance in regular daily existence.

Experience the vibe of being grounded in any circumstance.

Start to discharge your dread and outrage.

Comprehend your association with individuals, places, nature, and occasions in your general surroundings.

Progress further along your otherworldly way.

Start to help other people expertly.

Extend your insight into the arrangement of Reiki from a Japanese viewpoint.

Get individual continuous consideration and direction from your educator.

Have a place with a worldwide recuperating network, the International House of Reiki, and get every one of the advantages of the middle's incredible emotionally supportive networks. Okuden understudies are urged to resist for a base charge for proceeding with training purposes.

Third Degree Of Reiki: Shinpiden Self Treatment

Shinpiden centers on self-awareness and shows the understudy how to perform attunements. At this level, you move into finding increasingly about the puzzles of life. How you identify with yourself and the universe. This can be rehearsed for an amazing remainder and is constantly an individual practice, which can form into an expert showing practice on the off chance that you do want.

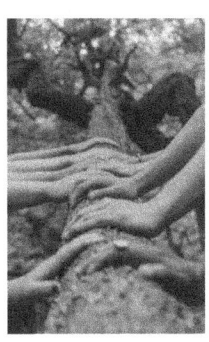

There are likewise more profound Japanese social and philosophical understandings that are instructed at each level, which will be clarified in more subtleties with the proper levels.

Shinpiden is the Japanese word for 'riddle lessons'. It is gone for Level II professionals or set up Reiki Masters who wish to proceed with their own voyage, an adventure that is progressing long after you complete the Shinpiden course. It is thusly not just about educating and is even appropriate for the individuals who wish to just build up their own Reiki practice and once in a while instruct people around them.

Self-strengthening is accomplished in Shinpiden through a solid enthusiastic association with the wellspring of Reiki.

It is additionally the consequence of the certainty you will feel because of your careful learning of Reiki – how it functions, what every one of the minor departures from Reiki really are, the place Reiki remains on the planet today, the Japanese

Shirusi (images) and Jumon (mantras) and their association with Japanese methods of reasoning and what the root of Reiki's otherworldly nature is.

One of the major focal points of this course is to take advantage of the feeling that you are, and consistently were, an incredible, brilliant light – this is accomplished by working with the fourth shirushi and jumon.

Advantages of Shinpiden Reiki:

Access a profound feeling of quietness.

Be sure as an instructor and professional.

Start to help other people expertly by instructing just as treating.

Get individual continuous consideration and direction from your instructor.

Have a place with a worldwide mending network, the International House of Reiki, and get every one of the advantages of the middle's incredible emotionally supportive networks.

Chapter 3: History Of Reiki

The system of Reiki contains a wide variety of different aspects which can be easy to overlook, as they can appear simple to those who don't know what they are seeing. However, these principles can be thought of as the foundation of the system that helps to bring awareness of Reiki to everyday life. These include meditation, regular Reiki practice sessions, embodying the symbols of Reiki, and understanding the true meaning of Reiki as well as how it came to be linked with atonement.

The principles that modern Reiki practices are based on are extremely ancient. The first person to rediscover them in modern times was a Japanese Buddhist monk named Dr. Mikao Usui. While teaching at a University in the late 1800s, Usui was asked by a student how Jesus Christ could have possibly performed the healing miracles that were attributed to him if he were not some type of higher being. This question stuck with Usui, and he eventually set out to answer it once and for all.

Usui's journey took him all around the world before eventually taking him back to the holy Koriyama Mountains in Japan. There he fasted and meditated for 21 days in hopes of reaching a higher state of consciousness that he believed would allow him to tap into the healing power that he was, by this point, certain resided somewhere within himself. On the morning of day 21, Usui started to become frustrated with his quest, as nothing he did appeared to be working. He was just getting ready to call it quits when he was suddenly filled with a supreme spiritual energy that entered his body through the top of his head, filling him with enlightenment as it did so. In addition to enlightenment, the energy also allowed Usui to tap into Reiki Ryhoho, or the ability to heal through touch.

Still reeling from everything he had learned, Usui returned home to his monastery but soon felt the urge to visit a local beggar camp in the slums of Kyoto.

He spent the next seven years in the slums treating a wide variety of illnesses with his new-found abilities and helping those who found themselves there to build a better life moving forward. Nevertheless, over time he found that the same people were returning to the area time and time again, regardless of what he did for them. When he asked why this was the case, he found out that they felt it was easier to go on begging than to take responsibility for getting things back on track once and for all.

Usui saw his Reiki as a type of spiritual practice, an opportunity for everyone he helped on their path to awakening their true nature, but he realized that many of the people he helped only saw him as a holistic alternative to more expensive medical treatment. As such, he altered his approach based on what he believed each patient or student needed. Some students would be shown various symbols to chant and meditate on while others might be taught to meditate on specific Reiki principles, and others might be tasked with sharing what they learned with others.

One of these in the last group was Dr. Chujiro Hayashi, a former naval officer and surgeon, who started studying with Usui in May of 1925. Hayashi was one of just 21 students who were tasked with passing on Usui's teachings prior to his death in 1926. After Usui's death, Hayashi opened a Reiki clinic which remained open for nearly 20 years. He also developed his own style of Reiki, which is largely the same as his mentor's. It uses the same lineage and energy pathways and is also the root of many of the more formal aspects of Reiki as it is taught today, including its hand positions and its practices, which are based on science. Hayashi's clinic soon proved to be extremely popular among the people, and word of it spread throughout all of Japan. This is also the point where many started to see Reiki as the primary path to healing as opposed to true spiritual enlightenment.

One of those who sought out help from the clinic was Hawayo Takata, a woman from Hawaii whose family was Japanese. In the early 1930s, her husband died, and she became quite ill with a disease that doctors proved unable to diagnose. She soon heard of Hayashi's clinic and decided to set out for Japan to see if there was anything to be done for her that wouldn't involve risky early twentieth-century exploratory surgery.

Once in Japan, she began receiving weekly treatments from Hayashi and quickly began to see improvements in both her physical and mental health. She was frankly amazed at the transformation she was seeing and asked Hayashi to teach her his secrets. He agreed, and she studied with him throughout 1936 and 1937, becoming one of just 13 students to whom he ultimately passed his techniques on to.

Takata was the first to bring modern Reiki practices to the west when she returned to Hawaii in 1938 and began to practice the technique herself at her own clinic. At first, she stuck to teaching just the first two levels of Reiki, but by the 1970s she started training other Reiki masters. She used storytelling to pass on the oral traditions of Reiki for more than 40 years. By the time of her death in 1980, she had trained more than 20 Reiki masters, and it is from them that modern Reiki practices have been passed on and codified.

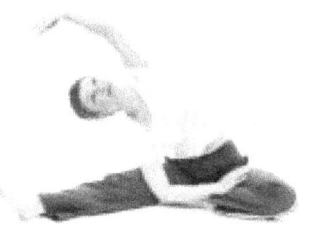

Usui Reiki became the most used and practiced in the world. It is important to know Usui Reiki, as it will make it easier to connect to its energy and ability to plan what's right for your well-being in life. Guidance from Reiki will help to make a difficult situation easier. It can bring an amazing change resulting in more positive results. Its use is available to everyone and not just on one person's intellect or spiritual growth.

There is nothing that is required for you to believe in to use it. Reiki is spiritual and comes from God, but it is not a religion. People find that using its principles, they gain religious experience, and not just learning what it is. It is important to live and promote harmony. Mikao Usui, recommends practicing certain easy ethical beliefs that will spread peace and harmony throughout the world.

When babies are born, they are all created with an abundance of energy. Always adapting, happy, filled with discovering, playing and never tired. As babies grow to adulthood, things change substantially along the way. They start to have worries, fears, and begin feeling tired, and physically and mentally depressed. Adults seem to find themselves angry, jealous, depressed and negative. Why does this happen? We are actually learning not to listen to what our bodies are telling us. We are told early in life to act a certain way and to react a certain way, usually by our parents. Also, other people can influence the way we may react.

All of these factors have a damaging effect on the energy that is given to us by God and the universe, which blocks our path. Reiki healing provides you with energy like it did when you were an infant to help you fight off the negativity in your body and fight diseases, sadness, anger, and depression.

Meaning and Definition of Reiki

From a spiritual perspective, "Rei" can be defined as the creation and progression of the universe, guided by a higher intelligence. Rei is a wisdom that penetrates and spreads into all that is spiritual and living. This wisdom teaches that creation leads to change from the beginning of galaxies to the everyday expansion of life. It is always here to help when we need it and to guide us through life.

The energy that is spiritual is referred to as "Ki", which means the energy that moves in everything that lives. It flows into all that lives such as plants, humans, and animals. If someone has high Ki, they will feel strength, confidence, and ready to challenge what life brings to them. When Ki is low, their weaknesses will consume them and leave them vulnerable to illnesses. Ki is received from breathing deeply, eating healthy food, getting plenty of sunshine and adequate sleep. Meditation and exercise will also increase Ki.

Reiki energy possesses its own intelligence that flows wherever it is needed to create healing conditions. A person's mind is never able to guide it, so it can't be controlled or misused by anyone. It is energy flowing through a person rather than from a physical condition and it is what is responsible for creating good health. If the force is interrupted for some reason, the organs and tissues will be negatively affected, which means low Ki can cause poor health and illnesses.

One of Ki's great attributes is that it reacts to a person's feelings and thoughts. It will flow with strength or can be weak depending on the strength of a person's mind. The more negative thoughts a person has, the more these thoughts are going to disrupt the flow of their Ki. It is estimated that nearly 98% of sickness is caused by a person's mind. A large part of the problem is with a person's unconscious mind because they are not aware of the problem. Therefore, it is much more difficult to solve.

The biggest benefit of Reiki healing is that it knows exactly where to go and what to do because a higher power guides it. When Reiki filters through an unhealthy space, it destroys and cleans any negativity trapped in the unconscious mind and body. This allows Ki to move freely through the body. The unhealthy physical organs and tissues are then properly nourished with Ki and start to flow in a healthy way, driving illness and weakness away from the body.

Reiki is becoming more and more popular because it is a healthy, non-invasive technique. Reiki will continue to be an important healing method as new alternative treatments are discovered.

Think of a beautiful pond with plants and flowers all around it. A simple path leads to the pond where you occasionally go to sit on a bench near the water. Ducks and birds come to swim and feed in the pond. One day you venture down the path to the water and see it is filled with algae and trash. The plants have been mowed haphazardly, and flowers are gone. The wildlife has disappeared, and the smell is horrible. Sadness and grief sets in.

Similarly, this is what happens when you have a healthy person who falls victim to negative energy. The negativity filters in, and over time, it creates unhappiness and an unhealthy way of life. This is like the energy surrounding the lake, which has been disconnected and needs to be revitalized.

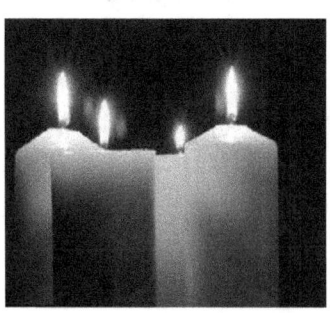

Chapter 4: Reiki: An Introduction

Reiki in Japanese means the 'Universal Life Energy'. The Reiki Healing System is a Japanese technique for relaxation and stress reduction that holistically affects the human system—body, mind, and spirit. Reiki reinforces healing and promotes personal development. There are Reiki principles to guide us through our spiritual undertaking; there are Reiki meditations to help us find back the inner power inherent in us; there are Reiki hands-on healing practices to attain a sense of wellbeing; there are Reiki symbols and incantations to balance the body and the mind; there are Reiki attunements to lift us up and help us regain our strength, health and peace of mind. To summarize, Reiki is the simplest path to make you feel connected with life.

The word Reiki in Japanese means 'spiritual energy'. Spiritual energy is in fact the perception of energy that is used in all the workings of Reiki practices.

Consequently, Reiki practitioners work with the energy of everything, believing that everything is composed of spiritual energy. It is aptly named 'Reiki'—pronounced ray-key—from the combination of two Japanese words Rei (Higher Power or God's Wisdom or Spiritual or Sacred) and Ki (Life-force or Energy). In combination, the Reiki Healing System is a spiritually guided Life-force Energy which is being used for stress reduction and relaxation to promote healing and also to treat various diseases and conditions. Reiki is also known as energy-healing, palm healing or hands-on healing. This healing technique uses various hand positions to attune and transfer energy by means of the palms to further healing.

Reiki can be learnt and practiced through a complete course, but the most ideal and strongly recommended way is to learn it directly from a skilled Reiki practitioner. It is also advised to experience a Reiki healing treatment on a regular basis. Reiki can be learned, practiced and experienced by anyone from childhood to old age. Reiki treatments are also extended to animals, birds and plants.

Origin of Reiki

The founder of Reiki—the Usui System of Reiki—was Dr Mikao Dr Usui, who developed the System based on his personal experiences in Japan in the early 1900s. Dr Usui developed Reiki through meditation, study, research and also through his knowledge and scholarship of the ancient Buddhist teachings. Dr Usui spent his entire life teaching and practicing this natural healing method which involved attunement to the energy using various hands positions laid upon significant parts of the receiver's body without however touching the body. The aim of the laying of hands system is to let Ki pass from the Practitioner's hands to the receiver's significant body parts. According to Dr Usui, hidden Life-force Energy flows through all living beings irrespective of whether they are humans, animals or plants. It is this Life-force Energy which causes living creatures to remain alive. If someone's Life-force Energy gets low, then they are more likely to become ill and/or feel stressed.

Reiki was taken from Japan and brought to the West 1937 by Hawayo Takata, a student of another great Reiki practitioner, Dr Chujiro Hayashi. According to her Reiki is around and within everything.

A more detailed account of Dr Mikao Dr Usui and his successors, Dr Chujiro Hayashi and Hawayo Takata, has been given in **The History of Reiki.**

Reiki: A Hands-on, Gentle Healing Process

It is believed that Life-force Energy originates from the Creator and, encompassing the whole of the Universe, flows incessantly in everything and in everyone. The abundance of Ki is limitless and can be accessed or used to create wellness and balance in the every sphere of life whether it is human, animal or plant-life.

The Reiki Healing System is a hands-on, gentle process of healing which balances the energy of the one who receives it. Using the hands, the skilled Reiki practitioner passes energy not only to their own body, but also to another person, animal or plant. When the energy gets through the receiver, they experience a sense of well-being, deep relaxation, comfort, and safety.

The natural healing method of Reiki is non-invasive, non-intrusive and non-manipulative since it is the receiver's body and not the giver or practitioner that determines where the Reiki goes and how much it receives. The Reiki Practitioner acts as a conduit or a vehicle through which the Universal Energy or the Life-force Energy flows. When Reiki practitioners place their hands, directing the energy on the receiver's body, they do not necessarily control that energy as it flows or assess how much of it is received by the patient. It is the acceptance and the willingness of the receiver of Reiki that determines the progress of the practitioner's healing process.

A Reiki treatment is generally one-hour long and is useful for specific healing or general relaxation. The client, generally in a lying down position, eased-up and relaxed, remains fully clothed at all times as the practitioner goes through a set healing process as agreed with their client prior to the treatment. Sex, age and condition are of no concern as the client's own body controls the process. During the treatment the body will only take the amount of energy that it requires. The Reiki practitioner places his/her hands on or just off the recipient's body with the intent that Ki (Energy) passes from the hands to the intended body part(s). The Ki is not pushed or forced from the hands; it is actually pulled out or extracted from them and through them by the recipient's body. Once the body senses the Ki, it receives it where it is most required. So, although the practitioner's hands may be placed on what is considered an 'area of need', there are more elements at play deciding on the direction and use of Ki. Reiki is therefore a treatment the frequency of which is individually tailored to the receiver's needs and conditions.

Reiki Complements On-going Treatments

As an established Reiki practitioner, I can give my assurances that Reiki has the power to help relieve many acute symptoms quite rapidly if received regularly and for longer hours. However, chronic problems will usually require Reiki treatments that can become more extensive. In such cases, the length of treatment will depend upon the energy needed to balance and revitalize the receiver's body, mind and spirit.

I also want to make it clear here that Reiki is not preconceived as a 'substitute' to standard medical treatments. Reiki is, most of the time, a complementary medicine which is meant to accompany, not to replace, standard medical practices. This is the reason why Reiki is today recognized by the Medical Community as a conventional or traditional medical approach. Hence, Reiki is almost never used to 'replace' ongoing medical or non-medical therapies of patients. The natural healing system of Reiki is wonderfully complementary and works effectively alongside the receiver's medical treatments and therapies.

Reiki - The Life-force Energy

We believe that Reiki nourishes every cell and organ of the living body. The Life-force Energy supports the vital functions of every living creature. When the flow of Life-force Energy is disrupted, the functions of the tissues and the organs of the body get diminished and sometimes even destroyed.

To put it in simpler words and looking at it from a personal angle, I will describe Reiki—the Life-force Energy—as that eternal 'Light' which is inherent in all of us from the moment we assume our shapes, whether human or animal. This 'light' goes out only when we finally leave our mortal shell. This immortal light, this brightness, is in reality our true nature—our Ultimate Source, our True Essence. However, as we grow older and progressively become tainted by the things of the world, this innate 'light' also gets slowly cloaked and obscured by the worldliness around us—

anxiety, fear, anger, attachments, greed, envy, jealousy.

As Life-force Energy is responsive to our feelings and thoughts, it is disrupted when we accept, consciously and unconsciously, negative feelings and thoughts either about ourselves or about our surroundings. All emotions and feelings affect our Life-force Energy. Once negative feelings take hold of us and of our thoughts, they attach and connect themselves to our energy field, thus disrupting our flow of Life-force Energy and diminishing the vital functions of the cells and organs of our body.

Consequently, the 'light' within us gets covered up so much that its brightness can no longer be seen with naked eyes. It is visible neither to ourselves nor to others who see us. And yet, even with our inherent light concealed, it continues to live within us, intense but camouflaged. The brightness is there; it's only that we cannot see it.

This is where Reiki comes in. Practicing the Reiki System of Healing helps slowly remove the layers of grime, stain and sootiness from our True Nature. Reiki helps remove from our 'inner light' the coatings of anxiety, fear, anger, attachments, greed, envy, jealousy and help us rediscover our authentic self.

The five very specific elements of Reiki, offered to us by the Reiki practitioner, help us heal our body, mind and spirit. These five elements are the Reiki precepts, the Reiki meditations, the Reiki hands-on healings, the Reiki symbols and the Reiki attunements.

And when all the muck, all the grubbiness is removed from our inner self, our true nature shines again; we become the Light, filling the space around us and enlightening those around us. We start feeling better, kindhearted, more compassionate and less prone to worries, anger and envy. When the inner self shines with inner light the world outside looks radiant and luminous too.

Reiki Heals Affected Parts of the Body and Mind

When a Reiki practitioner places his/her hand over a receiver's body, the Life-force Energy flows in the direction of the affected part(s) of the disrupted energy field and fill them up with positive energy. Reiki raises the energy field vibratory level in and around the physical body and especially in those parts which are affected by negative energies. With the rise of the vibratory level of the energy field, the negative energy breaks and falls apart. This is in fact the Reiki approach which straightens, clears, and heals the pathways of energy in affected minds and bodies and which allows the Life-force Energy to flow back naturally and in a healthy way. Again the objective here is to be willing to fully receive this miraculous natural therapy which works on the mind, the body and the spirit.

Reiki is Not a Religion

While the healing system of Reiki works wonderfully on the body, mind and spirit of the receiver and is essentially spiritual in nature, Reiki, however, is not a religion. One does not need to believe in any cultural system of behavior, in any order of existence or in any religion to be eligible to learn, use and practice Reiki. In fact, whether you believe or not, Reiki will still work on you and for you, because Reiki does not depend on any set of religious beliefs to function. Reiki has no dogma and there is nothing you must believe in order to learn, use and practice Reiki. The fact is that Reiki is not dependent on any belief at all and will bring its beneficial net result whether you believe in it or not. And the most wonderful truth about Reiki is that many people, from all walks of life and irrespective of cast creed or religion, find that practicing Reiki brings them closer and more in touch with the experience of their religion rather than having only a cerebral concept of their beliefs. They become more involved in their thinking, in their values and in their way of life. In short, these Reiki recipients ultimately come to have a better understanding of the essential and rational perception of their own religion.

Many of my Reiki students and recipients, who have undergone Reiki therapies with me, tell me that after their Reiki experience, their Reiki treatment or their Reiki class, they often have a sense of becoming more connected with their inner self, with the innermost core of their being. For me, this equals to reaching out to their inner spirituality.

Even while Reiki has nothing to do with religion, it still guides human beings to walk along a pathway where they can think, act and live in harmony with the Universe, with Nature and, at the end of the day, with themselves.

We will discuss in the next Chapter the ethical ideals of Reiki according to the priceless recommendations of Dr Mikao Usui. These Reiki Ideals offer suggestions about how to preserve, promote and disseminate Peace and Harmony across every culture in the world.

Chapter 5: Clearing Your Energy Field

Before you can perform a Reiki session, you have to clear your own energy field. If you do not clear your own energy field, most of the energy that is channeled will go toward healing and cleansing your own energy field and not that of your client.

The most important thing you will ever learn from a Reiki class is that you are to work on yourself first. The fact is that those who care for others tend to avoid taking care of themselves. The first rule of Reiki is that if you do not take care of yourself first, you cannot take care of others.

You also need to understand that it is up to you to heal you as it is up to the client to heal themselves. You see if a client comes in asking you to heal them you need to explain to them that you are just a vessel for the energy, they will be harnessing that energy and actually doing the healing themselves.

You need to make sure that you do not just jump into giving others Reiki, this needs to be performed on yourself on a regular basis. The more you do it, the better you will get and the more in tune with the energy you will become. I suggest you actually give yourself Reiki for at least 3-4 months before ever practicing on someone else.

You also need to understand that you're body needs to be as healthy as possible to be the best Reiki provider. If you are not eating healthy foods, drinking a ton of sugary drinks, not exercising and just not taking care of your body you will not be very successful at Reiki.

You need to also focus on your mental, emotional and spiritual state as well as the environment you live in. If you live in a stressful environment and try to work Reiki on others, you will find that it does not work because the energy will again try to heal you first.

So make sure you are taking the time out to meditate, create a calm place at home as well as in the office if you begin using Reiki on others.

Now as I said you need to practice Reiki regularly to clear your own energy field. You need to do this daily and not just when you remember to.

To do self Reiki, you need to start with a relaxing environment. Most people prefer to practice self Reiki first thing in the morning when they wake up and in the evening when they are going to bed.

Make sure you have a calm, relaxing environment, you can also have a soothing recording that you listen to while you practice Reiki. Next you need to make sure you are in a comfortable position and have a set plan. You need to work down your plan in the same pattern every day. It will look something like this:

Top of Head

Face

Neck

Chest

Abdomen

And work your way down as far as you want to go all the way to your feet if you would like. Then you will work backwards from your feet all the way back up to the top of your head or whatever starting point you have chosen.

You will take your hands and place them either on or right over the area you are working on. Hold them for a set length of time, two minutes seems to work great. You can use a small timer to track the time spent on each part of your body.

While you have your hands placed on or right above each area, focus on your breathing as well as whatever sensations you are feeling at the moment. If you finish one area but feel drawn to go back, repeat that area until you are comfortable removing your hands and moving on to the next area.

You want to do this for at least 3 to 4 months daily before ever practicing Reiki on someone else. Again you need to make sure you do this daily, I understand that there are times when you may not be able to fit in an entire session but some Reiki is better than no Reiki at all. If you can only focus on a few parts than make sure you focus on the ones you feel most drawn to. Either way, the Reiki energy is going to find the part of your body that it needs to work on at that moment.

While you are practicing Reiki on yourself, you will find that thoughts will come and go, allow them to but stay focused on your breathing, if a negative thought enters your mind, push it out and refocus. You may find that thoughts of what you have to accomplish that day or what bills need paid or even the random thought of what you need to purchase at the grocery store will try to creep into your mind, if it does let it pass, you can focus on those thoughts later but for now you need to be focused completely on balancing yourself.

As these thoughts enter your mind, just remind yourself that you are becoming balanced, you are healed and go back to focusing on your breath.

I have spoken to many people who have stated that in just one week of using self Reiki they have seen amazing changes in their lives. Some say that they just feel more positive and that they are able to think more clearly, others state they have become more productive and are much happier with life in general while still others say that in only a week they are seeing symptoms of health problems they have suffered with for years just disappear.

Before we go any farther, I want to make it clear that at no point should you quit taking any prescribed medications, it is okay to add some vitamins and minerals if a doctor says it is okay but until the doctor takes you off of your medications, continue taking them.

Chapter 6: Principles Of Reiki

Reiki is a way of life, and there are five fundamental principles to follow. Dr. Usui was disappointed to find that people who came to him for help did not go on to live better lives, despite seeing this fantastic revelation. He felt they should want to improve themselves and live more responsibly following healing through Reiki. Therefore, he created these five principles:

Just for Today- Do Not Worry

Worry is a useless emotion that causes illness and physically manifests itself (such as ulcers). Although people naturally worry, try not to worry for just for one day. You may well find that you are more relaxed, at peace and content.

Just for Today- Do not Anger

Anger is destructive and generally only damaging to the person experiencing it. It causes negative emotions and thoughts that spoil relationships and situations. Try for just one day to release all anger and just let it go. See how it feels to release your anger and live free of the aggression that goes with it.

Just for Today- Honor your Elders and Teachers

Your elders, teachers, and parents are generally people who want the best for you. These are people who want to see you safe, educated, and well. They deserve your respect; so do not let the few spoil it for the many. Most people in authority are there to help and support you, so remember for one day to honor your elders and teachers. Be thankful for them.

Just for Today- Earn Your Living Honestly

We are all different with unique gifts to offer the world. Do things honestly and respect your boss, the workplace, and the rules. Taking home a company pen may seem very insignificant, and no one would even know, but is it honest? Remember, it is essential to feel good about yourself, so be honest, respectful, and true to who you are.

Just for Today- Be Grateful for Everything

Be thankful, because there are so many things to be grateful for. Carry a notebook with yourself in which you write things you are thankful for. It is nearly impossible to be sad when you are thankful, what a compelling yet easy thing to be when you choose to be positive and happy through gratitude just for one day.

Chapter 7: Cleansing Your Energy

By now, you understand the powerful benefits of cleansing your energy through energy healing, but how do we go about doing this? If you are not ready to commit to meeting with an energy healer and getting on track that way, there are a multitude of simple things you can do at home to try and balance your energy on your own.

One of the strongest ways to accomplish this is through meditation. Like energy healing, meditation is nothing new, and you have probably come across this concept before if you are not already practicing. The concept is very simple. We must relax and focus our mind for the rest of our body, and our lives, to function properly. Our mind controls everything else, and so we must start here in our journey to overall wellness.

Meditation often calls upon energy from the earth to be imparted to the body to provide focus and insight. This energy surges throughout the body, pushing through energy blocks, resituating the mind where it should be. While there are many different types of meditation, asking for energy to enter your body is a great place to start.

Many offshoots of meditation offer benefit through passive means. That is, the mind has the ability to gather itself and focus by thinking of nothing at all. In fact, if your mind tends to wander, worry and get overwhelmed, there is a lot of benefit from meditating this way. Of course, as it does, energy will naturally flow in and out of you to create equilibrium with the environment around you. This process alone often leaves you feeling mentally acute and ready to handle the next task.

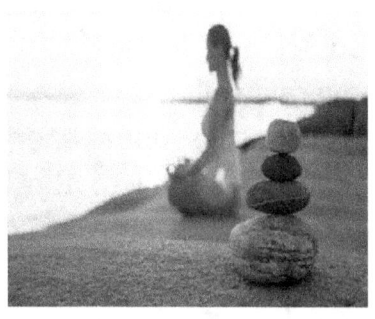

Energy healing takes meditation a step further. In this case, we do not passively meditate, hoping the universe will send us what we need. Instead, the idea of asking is imparted. In this asking, we sit silently, and simply imagine the energy we require entering our body. Many practitioners imagine it coming in through the very top of their head, traveling down the spine, and hitting every nerve on the way through. Imagine the feeling of energy flowing down every limb, descending to every finger and toe. Ask and you shall receive.

If meditation interests you, it is easy to get started. You will simply need a quiet room and yourself. Sit or lie down comfortably and focus on deep breathing. Let your breath steady and focus your mind on the ins and outs of your breathing. Let the stress of the day go and keep your focus. Once you have relaxed yourself a bit, decide how you would like to proceed. If you feel that honing in on your breath is energizing and fulfilling, keep that up. If you would like a little more, try asking for energy as the next step.

Practicing meditation daily, for about fifteen minutes can have amazing effects on your body and mind. If this is something you feel like adding to your daily routine, the last two chapters in this book are dedicated to guided meditation practice.

If meditation isn't in the cards, or you are looking for other simple things to do at home, look no further. There is a host of small, seemingly insignificant things that can be done on a regular basis to promote energy balance.

The first may seem obvious, you may not have realized its purpose. Most of us have partaken in a bath using bath salts. They are a popular Mother's Day gift as moms are usually characterized as stressed out. Salts are often infused with lavender and other essential oils to promote relaxation, but the salt by itself has amazing healing properties.

Salt is a polarizing substance. It draws water to itself. In the medical field, we are familiar with reducing salt to decrease fluid buildup that raises blood pressure and causes swelling, usually in the lower extremities. Water is a universal solvent, and everything, including toxins in the body, can be dissolved in this water. The salt draws this water out, toxins and all.

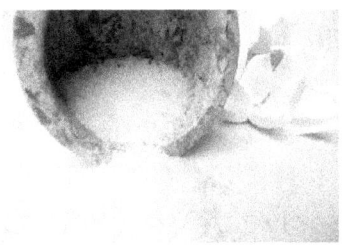

Salt is purifying in any form, and if you feel you don't have time for a daily salt bath, using it in the shower is another great way to incorporate it. Have a small container of bath salt or regular sea salt in the shower. As you wash away, take a little of the salt and run it over your skin. As you do, imagine negative energy and toxins leaving your body, as they are. Touching the salts to your chakra points has an even bigger benefit. More on chakras in the following chapters.

As discussed earlier, the mind has the power over everything else in the body. In that effort, we must do everything in our power to keep our mind calm and relaxed, so that it may move the body in a similar way. One great thing to do is to keep the spaces in which we live and work organized, clean and in good working order.

If you struggle to find things at home, making daily tasks just a little harder, you are unnecessarily stressing your brain. If your home is cluttered and your eye cannot pick a pleasant focal point, you are stressing your brain. By cleaning and streamlining your home or office space, you relax the brain and make it easier to do daily things, saving that extra energy for healing, or to increase your productivity.

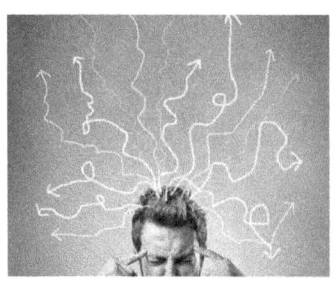

We have discussed many ways to gain extra energy from the earth, but often, this can actually be detrimental. For anyone who is anxious on a regular basis, getting more energy may actually be a problem. When the mind is on edge and anxious, there is likely too much energy, usually negative, flowing through the body. Anxious people often fidget and pace in an effort to burn some of that negative energy off. Using techniques like meditation, we can release negative energy from the body as well. Instead of asking for it, we can ask to release it through the soles of our feet.

If meditation isn't possible at any given moment, taking a few seconds to imagine that energy flowing out of us in moments of panic can have similar results. Tell the earth that this energy is too much to bear, and ask it to take it back. Imagine it flowing right out of you, releasing your muscle tension and reducing your jitters.

Exercise is another great way to relieve this negative energy. As anxious people often fidget, it shows that they are trying to burn the energy off naturally. Doing physical activity has the same effect. Walking, running or jogging creates a great release of energy from the whole body. Other exercises, like yoga and stretching, also promote the unblocking of energy channels, which can help release energy naturally as well.

Naturally, everybody is a little bit different and will require a different way to unwind and re-energize themselves. Often, different techniques can be used at different junctures in life to produce a good energy balance. Energies change, ebb and flow, and so we must use different tactics to resolve it. Most importantly, we must listen carefully to what our bodies are telling us, and give energy to areas that are lacking, and remove energy from areas that are overstimulated. Continue with techniques that bring you peace and energy, and forgo those that do not.

Chapter 8: Reiki Treatment

A REIKI therapy is awarded to a customer fully clothed, on a plinth and seated on a seat. The practitioner locations the hands of theirs on or above the customer. A treatment can last as much as an hour or often longer based on the treatment required. In the western world the professional will work with the standard hand positions then the total care is provided addressing the key organs of the body.

The fingers are put also gently on or perhaps above the body of the customer so there's absolutely no strain on the entire body, and that is perfect for dealing with any age as well as problems. The power is going to flow to exactly where it's required most (spiritually guided). The customer is going to experience a bright tingling sensation within the body. REIKI is an extremely calming and calming experience.

Every single individual's experience with REIKI is diverse, though the sensation of deep relaxation is experienced by most, a little experience a glowing radiance that passes through them and near them. Many people are able to drift off to sleep and some can have visions along with other mystical experiences. At the conclusion the person won't merely be relaxed but is going to have a balanced and positive outlook.

Reiki is a good healing method

REIKI is able to assist with a selection of complaints, to name some would be in, sinus, menstrual problems, PMT, respiratory problems, asthma, back problems, stomach discomfort, headaches, relieving pain, reducing stress, tension and many others.

REIKI helps in certain cases where individuals have experienced full healings that are established by healthcare assessments before as well as after the Reiki treatments. Nevertheless, while a few experienced miracles, they can't be assured. Reducing stress with a little improvement in one 's psychological and physical condition is what the majority of the experience.

REIKI should not be used rather than medical treatment, it ought to be used as a way and a compliment to become as well as remain healthy.

Reiki functions in union with consistent healthcare or maybe mental therapy. In case one has a psychological or medical condition, it's suggested that an individual see an authorized health care professional additionally to getting Reiki treatments. Reiki power works in harmony with any other types of healing, surgery, including drugs, psychological care or maybe some additional method of alternate care and can better the outcomes.

Though Reiki's power is spiritual in nature, Reiki isn't a religion. Practitioners aren't asked to change some spiritual or religious beliefs they might have. They're free to continue believing something they pick and therefore are urged to make their own decisions concerning the dynamics of the religious practices of theirs.

The Advantages Of Reiki Healing

It creates deep relaxation and also allows the body to release tension and stress.

It speeds up the bodies self healing capabilities.

It can help enhance sleep.

It lowers blood pressure.

Supports the immune system.

Might assist with intense (chronic problems and injuries) (asthma, headaches, eczema, etc.) and also might help with the breaking of addictions.

It is able to assist with the ease of soreness.

It's great the body rid itself of toxins.

It is able to help lower the unwanted side effects of medications and can allow the body to recuperate after chemotherapy and surgery.

It is able to boost energy levels as well as postpones the process of aging.

It increases the vibrational frequency of the entire body.

It's great with spiritual growth as well as mental clearing.

It is able to get rid of electricity blockages, regulate the power flow of the endocrine system bringing the body into synchronization and balance.

THE POSITIVES OF REIKI

1. Fosters Harmony and Balance

Reiki is able to prove to become a good tool in restoring your body 's balance on all of the amounts including physical, emotional, and mental, so all of the body parts might feature in total harmony. If a human body works harmoniously, it augments its organic healing capabilities which help all around health and health. In this regard, Reiki for babies is incredibly beneficial. It is able to contribute to the baby 's audio development and growth. Reiki can immediately target the root cause of the issue and rectify it rather than just relieving the symptoms.

2. Helps One Relax

Reiki could be remarkably peaceful as well as relaxing experience leaving an individual fully rejuvenated. Individuals who are stricken with emotional stress is able to attempt Reiki for nervousness as it might motivate a person to put out all negative feelings, anxiety, stress, and the tension to do a state of serenity, well being, and well being.

3. Dissolves Energy Blocks

Reiki therapy activates an understanding where one could be more conscious about the issues that appear to be robbing all of the peace and joy. It is able to help get rid of the big energy blocks in the type of negative thoughts or maybe self deprecating emotions to bring peace. One gets qualified to listen to their mind and body and take proper, mindful choices for the health of its. Being alert to your own needs is able to help you in accessing inner knowledge and wisdom which will help you cope with everyday stress in a much better manner.

4. Strengthens the Immunity

Frequent Reiki sessions are able to aid the body of yours to eliminate all of the dangerous toxins thus establishing the immune system. Many people stay in a continuous stress responsive battle function it upsets their body 's natural immunity and balance therefore giving them much more vulnerable to illnesses.

The bodies of theirs factually forget the best way to reinstate the balance. Reiki is able to have fun with a crucial part in telling the body to shift to rest/digest self healing condition that could help it to intensify the natural defense systems of its.

5. Improves Clarity and Focus of the Mind

Reiki is able to sustain you in staying centered in the current moment by handing over the car of the past regrets in addition to succeeding anxieties. It is able to heal mental and emotional injuries, lighten frustration and fears & enhance mental clarity and learning. It is able to fortify the ability of yours to deal with or handle situations as well as events that generally don't unfold based on one's preferred way.

6. Helps One Sleep Better

By stimulating the body to attain the natural balance of its as well as inner healing, Reiki enables an individual to sleep much better. When the mind of yours is for peace and free of worries and fears, you're certain to sleep very well. The greater an individual is in a relaxed room, the more she could be active and productive while not being exhausted stressed, or perhaps burnt out.

7. Treats Symptoms Linked with Cancer

Even though Reiki can't cure cancer, it might prove extremely successful in managing the symptoms regarding cancer as depression, fatigue, and pain. Reiki for cancer patients is usually one of the ways of supporting them deal with exhaustion, pain which often results after many cancer treatments. It can be utilized to strengthen them psychologically to fight cancer therefore improving the quality of theirs of life. Similarly, Reiki is able to bring considerable relief to individuals suffering from sciatica, arthritis, migraines, asthma.

8. Heals Inflammation as well as Infections

Reiki charged water may be a fantastic natural remedy to fix infections and inflammations. Emotional stress is able to give rise to many problems. Reiki not just lowers stress but additionally enhances the body 's immunity to battle infection. In this respect, Reiki during pregnancy could be especially useful. A pregnant female could be administered Reiki meetings to handle joint pain, infections that are common, and worry which generally happens during pregnancy.

9. Refines Personal Relationships

Reiki is able to help cure as well as advance individual relationships by rebuilding you psychologically. It is able to boost the capability of yours to relate and hook up to people on a profound level thus enhancing the relationships of yours. It is able to purify you of damaging feelings enabling you to realize inner peace which might, in turn, much better the capability of yours to freely love as well as open up to others therefore enabling friendships to flourish. You might start responding to life events and individuals in a supportive, trusting way instead of negatively.

10. Encourages Spiritual Growth

Reiki sessions operate an individual's self healing trip by way of individual development. It can help make a relationship with all the soul and endorses the characteristics of understanding, love, and validation. It can help an individual admit himself the way he's and also have compassion for other people.

Chapter 9: Reiki Lifestyle

There are many ways to incorporate Reiki into your lifestyle. Daily treatments on yourself are just a part of living Reiki and using it to guide you through your day. Whether it is diet, exercise, work, parenting, relationships, etc., Reiki can guide you and raise the vibration of your life.

Reiki and Food

We've touched on using Reiki with food, but now, it will be covered in a little more detail. When it comes to food, the quality of food you are eating is going to be very important. It is important for personal health, but it is also important for the cleanliness of the body.

As a Reiki practitioner, you are going to be channeling pure universal energy through you. As a conduit, you are going to want to remain healthy. If you are able to regularly eat clean foods, such as organic and unprocessed foods, you will remain a clearer channel for Reiki.

The clearer your body is the more sensitive your intuition and energy will become to the energy of your clients. This can make you a more effective energy worker.

Changing your eating habits or changing the kind of food you keep in your kitchen is going to be beneficial as you practice and learn Reiki.

It is so easy to come across unhealthy foods, overly processed foods, and mass-produced foods that are full of hormones, preservatives, and potentially harmful chemicals. In our society, those foods seem to be more easily accessible. Whether you are eating conventional foods or organic foods, including Reiki is a good way to get the most out of your food.

Being committed to a cleaner and healthier eating may not be easy, but if you are serious about being a Reiki practitioner, be more conscious about the foods and drinks that you are putting in your body.

That being said, Reiki energy can be used to raise the vibration of the food you eat. You can use these techniques on organic and conventional foods.

Using Reiki with your food is going to start when you are shopping for groceries. Whether at a Farmer's market, grocery store, natural food store, or supermarket, you can default to your intuition to find specific food items that will serve your higher good.

Call on Reiki energies as you are shopping with the intention of connecting with the food you want to buy.

Once the food is at home and in your kitchen, you can use either Reiki symbols, or a little Reiki energy to clear each food item as you put them away. This will help remove any residual energies the food items picked up from where they were grown, the store they were in, and on their travels to your home.

When preparing food to eat, using the Reiki distance symbol, or just a strong intent with Reiki energy can help you connect with the source of your food, i.e.

the farm it was grown on, the animal, or plant it came from.

Having that deeper connection with the energy of the source of your food is going to help imbue each meal with a deeper energetic connection. When you connect with your food energetically, you'll absorb more of the nutrients, clear away potentially harmful energies and toxins, but also deepen your own connection to life and energy.

Being a Reiki practitioner, having that strong connection to life and the source of energy is going to help you grow and progress as a healer.

Once a meal is prepared, use Reiki symbols or Reiki energy on the bowl or plate that you are eating from. Then serve yourself and use more Reiki energy over the entire meal. Also, charge your drinks with Reiki energy.

On a more serious note, if you are struggling with an eating disorder, Reiki can be beneficial in helping recover from that.

If eating is difficult for you in one way or another, trying performing Reiki on yourself before eating. Doing a quick session on yourself before a meal, or use Reiki symbols can help with the eating disorder or problems around eating.

Many people develop issues with eating, whether it is emotional eating or under eating, there are a lot of different manifestations of eating disorders. Some people associate food with negative experiences or abuse and it makes eating an uncomfortable experience.

This should never be the case! Eating should always be enjoyable. So, even if the act of eating is the problem and not the food itself, using Reiki on yourself and the food you are eating can help to overcome those disorders and those inhibitors.

Another option is to send Reiki to the time and place that you are going to be eating. That way once the meal begins, you can ease in with the Reiki energy guiding you.

You'll get the feel for how to use Reiki with your food. Food is our primary nourishment, so supplying that source of nourishment with the benefit of Reiki just strengthens our own nourishment and life force.

Working with energy is, in many ways, about connecting. Connecting to yourself, connecting to your spirit, and connecting to the universe and the energies of others. Bringing that connection into different aspects of your life, such as food and eating, is going to continue to bring your life fulfillment and satisfaction.

Reiki and Exercise

Movement is vital to life. Not only is movement required to keep our lymphatic system working, but movement prevents joint stiffness, muscle problems, and even bone problems.

Many individuals who don't exercise gain weight, lose feeling in extremities due to loss of circulation, have chronic pain from too much pressure being put on certain body parts while sitting or standing in the same positions, or in more severe cases, develop atrophied muscles.

Now, these are pretty extreme. It takes years of excessive not exercising to produce such results. However, movement and exercise are still vital.

In a lot of societies right now, movement and exercise aren't exactly encouraged. The majority of jobs are desk-based that require people to sit pretty much in a stationary position for 8 to 10 hours.

So much of our culture is based around computers, social media, phones, and even video games that after a day of work, or on days off, people lean more towards relaxing on the couch or at a desk rather than going out for physical activity.

Then there is the problem that many people have had where they had a negative experience with exercise. Whether it is because they were always picked last for sports on the playground, or they fell on a treadmill or were made fun of for their weight while out walking or running, a lot of people have had negative experiences with exercise.

So how can Reiki help?

Honestly, Reiki can help you be whoever you want to be!

If you have trouble exercising or are trying to motivate yourself to exercise more, put your workout clothes on and then give yourself a quick 10-minute treatment. After that, do some stretching, and then give yourself another ten-minute treatment. You can also use Reiki symbols as needed.

The distance symbol HSZSN that you learn in Level II Reiki is monumental in helping heal past traumas, insecurities, and bad experiences. If you use it while you are wearing your workout clothes, or before or after a light workout, it can help to heal those past experiences.

You can also use Reiki in manifesting motivation to exercise. Maybe you just feel too tired to exercise or have no motivation to actually do it! So write down your exercise goals on a piece of paper. Try to make them realistic. Maybe start with shorter-term goals in the beginning. Use Reiki symbols on the paper, or hold the paper in your hands and call for Reiki energy.

Keep that paper in your pocket anytime you do anything physical, whether it is a simple walk or a more rigorous workout routine.

You might not have any trouble getting yourself to exercise, but seeking to reach a specific goal with exercise, such as weight loss. Reiki energy and Reiki symbols can help to promote such a goal.

If weight loss is your goal for workouts, balancing symbol SHK that you learn in Level II Reiki is also a great symbol to promote weight loss. Use the symbol specifically on the areas of the body that you would like to lose weight from before you start your workout routine.

If you aren't Attuned to Level II, hold your hands over a specific area of the body you would like to lose weight from and let Reiki flow there before you start a workout.

Another way to incorporate Reiki into exercise to make the most of it is, if you already have a workout routine, trying having Reiki energy flow through the entire workout. Almost like a combo workout and self-treatment session.

This can be done for rigorous workouts or for a simple and easy walk. Either way, intending that you receive Reiki for the duration of the workout or exercise will really take it to the next level.

You might lose weight faster, get toned muscles faster, find your endurance increasing, having more motivation to exercise, or just simply feeling more connected to your own body and skin.

Getting into a good exercise routine and making healthy habits out of exercise is going to take a little time. Reiki can help motivate you and help you reach your exercise goals. It can also help you overcome any adversities you have in regards to exercise.

Reiki and Water

Water and hydration are such an important part of the human existence, that it deserves additional attention away from food.

There are plenty of studies to show how water molecules are impacted by energy vibes. It was touched on previously how positive words, thoughts, and feelings alter the molecular structure of water the same way negative thoughts, words, and feelings do.

Everyone should be drinking water daily. More than that, we use water to wash our hands, wash our dishes, bath our bodies, water our plants, etc. There are endless uses for water around the house.

Reiki energy can be used to improve water quality and give it healing, balancing power. With a glass of water that you intone a Reiki symbol into or channel Reiki energy into, the taste of the water changes. Even if ever so subtly.

Using Reiki energy on the water meant for your plants and gardens can help promote healthy and abundant plant growth.

Washing your hands in Reiki treated water will help keep your hands a pure and clean channel for healing yourself and clients.

Start treating the water that you drink, water plants with, and wash your hands with Reiki energy. You might be pleasantly surprised in the differences you start to notice.

Reiki can be used to turn water into a healing elixir. By drinking Reiki treated water, those treated molecules can change the energy vibration of the rest of the water molecules in your body!

The origin of life is in water, from the very oceans of our planet. This makes water a powerful source of life energy. Even if it is coming from a tap, that water is still connected back to the source. Therefore, using Reiki on the water is going to increase your connection to life energy and improve your overall vibration.

Reiki Blessings

You can also start to use Reiki in blessings. Blessings don't have to be major or formal, but add a little Reiki to them and start to see how the environment around you improves.

If you are a plant owner or gardener, use Reiki to bless seeds or potted plants by channeling Reiki energy into the seeds as you hold them, or by putting your hands on either side of a plant pot. You can also use Reiki symbols on seeds and pots.

Or you can bless an entire garden with Reiki. If you are a first-time gardener or starting something new, like a vegetable garden, offering some Reiki energy can help ensure healthy plant growth.

If you are moving into a new house or apartment, blessing each room with Reiki before moving in can ensure a happy stay in the home. Channel energy directly into the room, or use Reiki symbols to beam the energy into the rooms. If you are buying a house or moving into an apartment with a romantic partner for the first time, use Reiki to bless the space for harmonious coexistence.

Maybe you have a job interview coming up and want to ensure that it goes smoothly. Send Reiki to the time and place of the interview, blessing it with balancing energy and success. The distance symbol learned in Level II Reiki is the best method for sending Reiki energy through time and space.

Small Reiki blessings can be used in all kinds of scenarios throughout the day. Getting in the habit of using Reiki energy during your daily activities will literally transform the environment around you. The balancing energy will go where it needs to and as you work on yourself too, you will start to attract the types of things into your life that you resonate with.

So, working on yourself while adding small Reiki blessings into your own world, you start to create the world that you truly want for yourself. The idea of blessings may seem odd or like a religious concept.

In this case, blessings are simply adding positive or balanced energy to situations or aspects of your life. Reiki has innumerable uses when it is applied to seemingly menial daily activities and tasks.

The more you practice, the more it will become a habit for you to call on Reiki every day. This is how you start truly living Reiki.

Reiki and the World

Using Reiki to change your own environment and the direct world around you is great for your personal life and personal abundance and health. However, since Reiki can be sent across time and space, sometimes, using it on a larger scale can be helpful.

For example, if there is a natural disaster in part of the world, setting aside time to send Reiki energy to that area of the world and to the relief efforts can lend a helping hand. It can also improve the mood and overall conditions of life in areas that have been harmed by natural disasters.

A single Reiki practitioner won't have the power to completely alter the course of an entire natural disaster relief effort. However, every little bit helps, and if other Reiki practitioners are pitching in, which they should be, then more energy will keep getting sent to that area.

Reiki energy can be sent into specific situations as well. Consider political situations or areas of conflict and war in the world. By sending Reiki energy into those situations, the balancing and healing process begins. While one practitioner may not be able to change an entire political situation or end a war, as long as practitioners are sending out the healing energy into these situations, change will happen. Change in the form of balance and healing.

Maybe there is an area of the world that is suffering from a drought or crop blight. While in our modern society that might not seem like such a big deal, but droughts and blights and other types of famines can and do still occur. Their impact may be localized, but it is still an impact.

Reiki energy can be used to try and relieve the impact of such blights. Reiki can help rebalance the environment to bring rain. It can rebalance soil for nutrients. Reiki can also provide balance to an ecosystem to prevent an overpopulation of crop pests.

Most Reiki practitioners who are committed to living the Reiki lifestyle and being Reiki healers will take notice of global unrest, whether it be natural or human-based, and lend Reiki energy as needed.

Healers tend to be community-oriented. If there is a disruption in your community, offering Reiki energy can help a situation. This could be as simple as a water main break or more serious in the event of a missing child. Even from a distance, providing Reiki energy can promote a resolution or solution. In the least, it can provide balance, clarity, and relax tensions.

In a closer to a home setting, say you have a tree in your yard that is in bad health or diseased. Supplying that tree with Reiki energy can help heal the wound or disease and bring it back into a healthy state.

Reiki energy is a powerful force. It exists through the entire universe. While it is primarily used for treating yourself and other people with healing sessions, Reiki isn't limited to just treatments.

In everyday life, Reiki can be used in food, to help with exercise, and to make healing elixirs. Reiki can be used to help global situations like natural disasters, wars, and political unrest. It can work in communities to solve smaller problems and even in your physical environment. You can also include Reiki in everyday tasks and activities to change the very frequency of the world you live in!

The uses for Reiki are innumerable. To start living the Reiki lifestyle, just take a moment to think of all the times and situations in any given day that you could add some Reiki energy in order to improve that task.

Reiki can be used on people, animals, inanimate objects, and plants. Reiki can be used on manmade and natural objects. Reiki energy can be sent through time and space and to specific situations.

The more you incorporate Reiki into your everyday life, the better you will feel. The more at home you will feel in your own environment. This will lead to a more balanced and satisfactory life.

Chapter 10: Life With Three Eyes

Life with an open Third Eye is very different to life with just the "standard issue" two. In this final chapter we'll take a look at some of the changes – and the new experiences and sensations that you will begin to see appearing in your life.

An Eye in the Back of Your Head?

You may have heard the saying "they must have eyes in the back of their head" and when you have opened your Third Eye you may begin to see and experience the world in a whole new way. Intuitive abilities are often the first to develop as the complex relationship between our conscious and sub-conscious mind becomes more attuned. Our sub-conscious is the repository of all of our experience – many would argue both in this life and previous ones. When you have activated your Third Eye you have far greater access to this side of yourself and soon you'll see patterns in life, in events and in circumstances around and you'll be much quicker at seeing the most likely outcome of situations. Gradually this will build into truly "clairvoyant" abilities – the abilities to see so clearly that it seems – and may well be – that you can predict the future.

Meet The Ancestors

As your Third Eye heals and develops there is also a strong likelihood that your connection to, and ability to communicate with, the world of spirit will increase dramatically. We all have spirit guides and we are all influenced by the spirit world continuously. This normally manifests in most peoples' lives as simply being in the right place at the right time, or noticing some "uncanny" coincidences, which lead them to make a specific decision. With an active, healthy and fully functioning Third Eye, this communication will become more two-way and you may find that spirits will speak to you directly. This is often apparent at first, when you begin to sense close friends or family members who have passed away. In time, this sense will develop to include those who gather around other people, including complete strangers.

Strange Vibrations

Many people develop these in the early stages of de-calcifying the Pineal Gland and opening their Third Eye. The most common sensations are a strong tingling in the area at the center of the forehead, where the Third Eye is traditionally depicted. For some this is a light, tickling sensation as if being brushed with a feather. For others, the feeling is of a constant, pressure or touch. In a minority of cases headaches or even migraines can occur. This is rare but does happen on occasion; headaches will pass in a few days, usually become less strong over that period. These sensations are widely documented and no cause for concern but simply a natural part of the process. The light tingling or touching sensation will usually pass after a few weeks – or at least become so familiar that it goes unnoticed.

Some individuals find that during periods of insight, medium-ship or clairvoyance they notice or experience the sensation again. Many individuals with an active Third Eye take this to be an indication that there is a need to use the abilities (clairvoyance, medium-ship or spirit contact) as and when the sensation returns.

Living with the Dead

Death is not an end, simply a transition and a natural part of our spiritual journey.

It's an inevitable part of opening your Third Eye that you will begin experience more contact with the world of spirit. In the early days after opening your Third Eye this contact will most often come in the form of dreams. Lost relatives or friends may appear in your dreams in a more vivid way than they have in the past. Conversations with them will seem more "real" in dreams and this is no coincidence! Listen carefully to what they say and be sure to consider any advice they give you. While spirits of all kinds have a more far-reaching view of our own world and lives, don't assume you must take all advice! Certainly the beings you find yourself in contact with are well informed but it's important to learn (or remember) to act using your own intellect and initiative and not come to rely on otherworldly advice.

Encountering spirits in dreams is common in the early stages of developing your Third Eye, but encountering them in the waking world is not uncommon and is increasingly likely as you develop your skills. Thanks to Hollywood, our impression of "ghosts" is largely negative and may leave you fearful for your safety.

In reality, this impression is flawed; you're more likely to come to physical harm from a real person, in the real physical world, than you are from any spirit contacts you make. The physical realm is not the natural realm of spirit – it's yours! Remember this, and with this in mind, be aware that you can always ask unwanted, unwelcome or unhelpful spirits to leave. They have little choice but to do as you request and your intention is important here. Mean what you say and say what you mean when dealing with spirits of all kind. This works with people in our physical lives as well!

Heightened Sensitivity

This is an often overlooked issue for people dealing with their new skills. With an active, healthy Third Eye you will very quickly become more intuitive and extremely open to the emotions of the people around you. This can include complete strangers as you pass them on the street. Emotions are big things; they can be great and they can be terrible. Opening yourself up to them can leave you feeling drained and exhausted. You will certainly find that you'll be unwilling to spend time around those who emanate negative emotions and your sense of empathy will expand rapidly as you open your Third Eye. Empathy should not be confused with sympathy – you will feel what the person you are connecting with feels as if the feelings were your own.

As you take your first steps working with the Third Eye the best advice is to avoid those people or situations in which you are exposed to negative emotions. These will drain your energy and can leave you unable to work effectively with your Third Eye or enjoy the benefits of using it. However, as you become more experienced in life with three eyes, consider the benefits that your new "powers" can offer others. An important part of our spiritual growth is related to the way we interact with the world around us and, particularly, the way in which our actions to others are conducted. Using your "powers" or abilities to benefit only you will lead you to becoming small, narrow minded and selfish, which will ultimately destroy those powers! Learn to be strong and use your abilities of empathy to help, to heal and to benefit those around you. Importantly, remember to take time for yourself; walk in the woods and mountains alone, meditate, swim, and daydream. Whatever "re-charges" your batteries, ensure you make as much time for this as anything else; this will help to ensure that you have the reserves of strength to use your skills to their best effect.

Getting, or Staying, Physical

Many people have neglected their Third Eye for so long that opening it can be an astounding experience. It can become, almost, an obsession but remember that while it is massively important to your spiritual development you are not, as yet, pure spirit. We have real, urgent, physical needs in life; they're simple and include staying fit and healthy, eating well and socializing. All of these activities should be considered as cornerstones of your life. With an open Third Eye it is likely that you'll find that you are actually keen to eat and live healthily; go with that feeling! Learn to balance your physical, emotional and spiritual needs equally in life and make time for all three.

New Friends and Old

As your spiritual journey progresses you may find that some people in your life don't fit anymore. Don't be afraid of this – we all outgrow people from time to time. As your psychic and spiritual path progresses it's likely that you'll seek out new opportunities for learning and development and these will also bring new contacts into your life. Don't be afraid to let go of the past and explore the future in all areas of your life. This doesn't mean you should drop friends or associates lightly – you may have a deep bond with many of them and they may contribute to who you are in ways that you have yet to discover. However, if some contacts are lost as part of your journey learn to accept that this is part of the process.

Patience, Patience, Patience

Finally, be patient as you await the opening of your Third Eye. The steps and advice in this book will help to make the process real and viable but it can take more time for some than it can for others. For those already with a deeper spiritual awareness or natural clairvoyance the process can be rapid – days, weeks or a couple of months. For some, it can be lengthier, with progress and delays on the way. Remember to be patient and to persevere; you may need to make many changes in your life as your skills develop and some of these can take time and effort to achieve. The more times you try, the greater your chance of success and don't, whatever you do, be put off by occasional failures – pick yourself up and start again. You will get there!

Chapter 11: History Of Reiki

Many think that Mikao Usui or Usui Sensei as he is respectfully alluded to, was the maker of Reiki and that the word Reiki applies just to the mending methodology he founded and created. However, when looking into the cause of Reiki as a recuperating methodology, we find that before Usui Sensei built up his style of Reiki, there were already four different styles of Reiki healing that were being practiced in Japan. This data originates from Hiroshi Doi Sensei and from Toshitaka Mochizuki Sensei, two Japanese Reiki scientists.

Other Reiki recuperating procedures that were being used before Usui's strategy were:

Mataji Kawakami made Reiki Ryoho

Reikan Tonetsu Ryoho made by Reikaku Ishinuki

Senshinryu Reiki Ryoho made by Kogetsu Matsubara

Seido Reishojutsu made by Reisen Oyama

In any case, as a result of the conditions created during the World War II, different types of Reiki remained generally obscure and Usui Reiki developed to be the dominating type of Reiki practiced around the world.

Usui Reiki

Dr. Mikao Usui was born in 1865 to a wealthy Buddhist family. His parents provided a well-balanced education for him compared to what was found at the time. He studied in a Buddhist monastery where he was taught martial arts, swordsmanship and the Japanese form of Chi Kung known as Kiko.

Much later, Dr. Usui was teaching in a Christian seminary and one of his students questioned his belief in Jesus' healing and if he did believe, when were they (the students) going to be taught how to heal?

A gentleman through and through, when Usui realized that he could not teach his students any healing technique, he embarked on a journey of self-realization. He committed himself to studying how he felt Jesus, Buddha, and other religious figureheads were able to heal their followers. He traveled widely, learned different languages and learned different healing systems of all sorts.

He sought to find a way or methodology of healing that would be acceptable to everyone regardless of religion. He wanted all to be able to access his healing method, so he yearned for one that was not connected to any religious belief.

He ended up in a Buddhist monastery where the Abbot advised him to meditate on the answers he sought. This prompted him into starting a 21-day fasting retreat. It was his own personal rediscovery course in a cave in Mount Kurama.

At the end of the intense prayer, fasting, and meditation, Usui experienced an extraordinary event. He was apparently struck by a great light. In his trance, he saw the ancient Sanskrit symbols that had helped him develop the system of healing that he was hoping to invent. He received spiritual empowerment and an Awakening. Despite going without food 21 days, he was surprisingly energetic when he woke from his trance. He ran down the mountain. In his haste, he struck his foot against a stone. As he reached down to touch it, he discovered that the bleeding had stopped and there was not any pain. He would later heal the Abbot of his arthritis and a little girl, of her toothache. Such was the birth of Usui Reiki healing technique.

After his spiritual Awakening on Mount Kurama, Usui established his first healing clinic and school in Tokyo in 1922 and was soon well known for his healing miracles. He spent long years healing people in Japan before he passed on his knowledge to Dr. Chujiro Hayashi who was a Naval commander at the time.

Before his death, he had taught several Reiki Masters including Dr. Hayashi to ensure that his knowledge and method of healing would endure the test of time. He also encouraged Dr. Hayashi to open his own Reiki Clinic. Usui Sensei later died in 1926 after suffering a massive stroke.

Motivated by Usui Sensei's request to set up his own clinic, Hayashi Sensei started a school and clinic called Hayashi Reiki Kenkyukai (Institute). Hayashi made pivotal changes to the way Reiki teaching was being done at the time. These changes require that the client lie down during treatment instead of seating in a chair that Usui practiced. He also created a more effective way of performing attunements.

He also developed a new system of teaching Reiki where Reiki 1&2 were taught together as a five-day seminar. Dr. Hayaki is also credited with introducing hand positions to completely cover the body and give a better overall flow of energy to every part of the body. He also provided additional positions to be used for certain specific conditions.

In 1935, a Japanese-American woman named Hawayo Takata who was visiting relatives in Japan came to his clinic to treat a serious ailment. She was so impressed by the Reiki healing method that she requested to learn under Hayaki until he reluctantly agreed.

The following is a summary of Takata Sensei's version of her early years leading up to her contact with Reiki at the Hayashi clinic. It comes from an interview that appeared in The (San Mateo) Times, May 17, 1975 titled "Mrs. Takata Opens Minds to Reiki" by Vera Graham:

"She stated that she was born on December 24th, 1900, on the island of Kauai, Hawaii. Her parents were Japanese immigrants and her father worked in the sugar cane fields. She eventually married the bookkeeper of the plantation where she was employed. His name was Saichi Takata and they had two daughters. In October 1930, Saichi died at the age of 34, leaving Mrs. Takata to raise their two children.

In order to provide for her family, she had to work very hard with little rest. After five years she developed severe abdominal pain and a lung condition, and she had a nervous breakdown. Soon after this, one of her sisters died and it was her responsibility to travel to Japan, where her parents had resettled to deliver the news.

She also felt she could receive help for her health issues in Japan.

After informing her parents and attending the funeral, she entered a hospital and stated that she was diagnosed with a tumor, gallstones, appendicitis, and asthma. She was told to prepare for an operation but opted to visit Hayashi Sensei's clinic instead.

Mrs. Takata was unfamiliar with Reiki but was impressed that the diagnosis of Reiki practitioners at the clinic closely matched the doctor's at the hospital. She began receiving treatments. Two Reiki practitioners would treat her each day. The heat from their hands was so strong, she said, that she thought they were secretly using some kind of equipment. Seeing the large sleeves of the Japanese kimono worn by one, she thought she had found the secret place of concealment. Grabbing his sleeves one day she startled the practitioner, but, of course, found nothing. When she explained what she was doing, he began to laugh and then told her about Reiki and how it worked.

Mrs. Takata got progressively better and in four months was completely healed. She wanted to learn Reiki for herself. In the spring of 1936, she received First Degree Reiki from Dr. Hayashi. She then worked with him for a year and received Second Degree Reiki. Mrs. Takata returned to Hawaii in 1937, followed shortly thereafter by Hayashi Sensei, who came to help establish Reiki there, and his daughter. In February 1938, Hayashi Sensei initiated Hawayo Takata as a Reiki Master".

Hawayo Takata returned to Hawaii in 1937 and established the first Reiki clinic in the West and continued to teach and heal others. She traveled widely all over America and Canada imparting the Reiki knowledge to many as she traveled.

Chapter 12: The Reiki Healing Techniques

Karuna Reiki

Karuna is a word that means any action that helps to diminish other people's suffering. In Sanskrit, Karuna means "compassionate action." The Karuna system of Reiki is a technique developed by William L. Rand when he used the symbols channeled by other Reiki Masters like Kellie-Ray Marine, Pat Courtney, Marla Abraham, and Marcy Miller. Rand found the symbols to be very valuable, but he felt that they still had a lot of potential locked deep within them. He used guided meditation to become attuned with the symbols to unlock their full potential, and he called this new Reiki technique Karuna.

Karuna Reiki's energy is applied with more focus and also works on all energy bodies simultaneously. People who receive attunement from their Reiki teacher only when they have become qualified Reiki practitioners. They often need to report to their Spirit Guides, Angels, and their

Higher Self, and then afterwards they feel their presences at times.

Benefits of Karuna Reiki

Non-invasive

Helps heal unconscious patterns/habits

Can help with sleeping problems

Can help easy panic attacks, fatigue, and muscle pain

Can help with the manifestation of personal goals

Helps pull out the negative energy, or blockages in your ki flow and helps release pain

Can also help ease emotional pain

Does not require you to convert into another religion

Heals the body on a cellular level

Helps you deal with past-life issues

Helps you fix communication problems

Helps you deal with co-dependency

Helps mend relationships and makes them better

Helps you be more mindful and in the moment

Helps you shatter your denial habits

Helps with self-image problems\

Improves learning and promote clarity of the mind

Sekhem or Seichim Reiki

Sekhem is an ancient Egyptian word that means "Universal Energy or Power", roughly translate as "Power of Powers". Sekhem in Egyptian hieroglyphs is symbolized by the scepter, and it represents the connection between Heaven and Earth.

Sekhem healing energy can help accelerate your spiritual growth, but most importantly, it can open communication channels with your "higher self" and with the "All That Is", which can mean different things to different faiths (the Cosmic Universe, the Divine Creator, the Soul of Souls, etc.) There are no other known energy system that can compare with the high vibrational energy of Sekhem, nor does any other energy work at a deeper soul level.

Sekhem Reiki promotes being more responsible for your life. It also allows you to heal, and it helps your personality and spirituality, so you can find your soul's purpose and unlock your full potential.

Benefits of Sekhem or Seichim Reiki

Fast physical, spiritual, and emotional healing

Quickens the neverending process of spiritual development and enlightenment

Assists in the manifestation of goals

Improves your "inner sight" and your ability to sense the energy around you

Increases your "feeling of being alive" by making you more aware of the present

Increases your self-awareness and your relationships with others

Western Reiki

Almost all of the Reiki practiced in Japan is Westernized Reiki, which is quite ironic considering that Reiki originated from Japan. There was a time when people thought that there were no more any legitimate Reiki practitioners left in Japan. That is why when Reiki was reintroduced into the country, the Japanese people who wished to learn it had to visit North America to get tutelage. However, the successors of Usui-sensei have always been in Japan.

First of all, there's the Usui Reiki Ryoho Gakkai, the organization that was founded by Mikao Usui himself. This group is composed mostly of the original Masters that were trained by Usui. The reason why this organization has been almost unknown to the world was because the members chose to remain a closed group, but recently they decided to open up their doors for new members.

There are also the surviving students of Chujiro Hayashi, which was one of the prominent students of Mikao Usui. One of his students was Hawayo Takata, who was believed to be the person who introduced Reiki to the Western hemisphere.

Benefits of Western Reiki

Promotes acceptance of oneself

Can help minimize pain and discomfort; can actually be used to aid in natural childbirth

Can assist a dying person's soul transcend peacefully to the afterlife

Can aid in being more mindful of one's thoughts and physical feelings
Can help uncover hidden emotions so they can be easily healed
Can balance the chakras in the body
Can be used to complement other medical treatments safely
No need to convert to other religions
Non-invasive and gentle healing
Provides natural pain relief
Promotes deep relaxation and helps cure sleeping disorders
Promotes wholistic health and well-being
Is safe for use by pregnant women
Hastens the recovery from surgery sickness, and eases labor pains
Can help ease and eliminate stress

Chapter 13: Introduction To The Guided Meditations

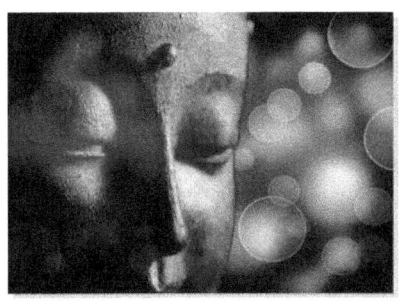

Guided meditation is when you do a meditation usually with an experienced mediator who guides you through your meditation with his voice. He will indicate what you have to do at every moment of your meditation. Most guided meditations have music playing in the background to help you get into the mood of meditation which will be a state of tranquility.

There are some guided meditations that have a specific purpose such as to relieve stress or to generate compassion. Yet, others are there to help you observe your thoughts or take control of them.

Starting meditation can be overwhelming at first, but it can help you to reduce frustration while having someone there to guide you through your first few sessions.

The goal of guided meditations is to make it to where you do not need any external help in the end. Meditation is supposed to be a cold space in your mind where you are alone with your thoughts. Be aware, that in the beginning, meditation is not easy and may seem boring, but that is why you have to take baby steps to get to your final goal.

It is recommended that after you get to at least 20 minutes of guided meditation, you should start trying to meditate on your own.

During your guided phase, you should start with 1 minute of meditation and move up. Every day is going to increase until you hit 20 minutes which is when you should begin to feel comfortable enough to meditate on your own.

When you meditate on your own, you need to use a timer to control your meditation. Figure out what type of meditation you want to do and do it without guidance.

Calming meditation: Whenever you feel anxious or agitated, this meditation can help you to calm your body and your mind. Breathe slowly and repeat your mantra to yourself that will help you to bring feelings of well-being and deeper inner peace. Become aware of your breathing and allow your breath to fall freely and rhythmically.

Inner peace meditation: Uplifting meditations are meant to help you fall into a zone of peacefulness. Focus on every breath that you take and release. You should start to feel yourself moving towards a place of inner pace. In the event that you want to cultivate a specific virtue, you should write it down and place it where you will see it every day.

Body scan meditation: With body scan meditation, you will become aware of various parts of your body and become attuned to how each part feels without judgment. You are supposed to cultivate an open and compassionate attitude about your body. You may also focus on wider parts of your body or narrow it down to specific regions. In order to use body scan meditation, you will lie down and direct your attention over each part of your body one at a time.

Loving-kindness meditation: Sit quietly with your eyes closed and your muscles relaxed as you take deep breaths. You should imagine your entire body and feel the perfect love for yourself. Thank yourself for everything that you are and that you know. Repeat several reassuring and positive phrases to yourself. Allow yourself to focus on the positivity flowing around you. If you stray, redirect your attention back to what you are doing.

Breathing meditation: Choose a quiet place to meditate. Sit somewhere where you do not allow yourself to get distracted nor you will become sleepy. Get rid of all distractions and close your eyes. Breathe naturally without trying to control your breathing; you should become aware of the sensations you feel as the air enters your body and leaves. Concentrate on these feelings and nothing else.

Walking meditation: Find somewhere where you feel safe to walk. While you are meditating, you should not become too deep in your meditation that you place yourself in danger. Pay attention to your feet as they hit the ground while you keep the same pace. Allow yourself to think about the goals that you want to accomplish and imagine your stress falling to the ground each time your foot hits the ground.

Focused attention meditation: Focus all of your attention on one thing such as what your goals are. You will need to find a quiet place and visualize what your goal is. The more you focus on your goal, the stronger it will become, which means that the less there will be to distract you from your goals. Just remember that the stronger your visualization is, the more likely you will reach your goal.

Zen meditation: With Zen meditation, you will sit on the floor with your legs crossed, arms in rested position, and hands formed in oval. Focus on your breathing and count how many times you breathe in and how many times you breathe out. You need to also focus on your posture. Most people practice Zen in the lotus position.

Vipassana meditation: Vipassana is practiced like Zen but the difference is that you have to develop a sense of concentration by using a practice known as samatha. Once again, this is usually done by becoming aware of your breathing. Focus on every moment that passes and what you are doing in that moment. You may notice that there are small changes to your breathing that you have never noticed before—like how your abdomen rises and falls or how the air feels as it enters your nose or passes over your lips.

Mantra meditation: This is quite easy to do. You will find a mantra that you want to instill in your mind and you will repeat it as you meditate. The mantra meditation helps you focus on your goals or helps you to bring more positivity into your life.

Transcendental meditation: This meditation type is not usually taught. You will do transcendental meditation twice a day. It is similar to mantra meditation, but you will not be making up your own mantra; you will be assigned one that is based on your age, gender, and where you are in life. This type of meditation has to be learned from someone who is licensed to teach it.

Chapter 14: The Eastern Version

Dr Usui was born on August 15th 1865 in the village of Yago in the Yamagata district of Gifu prefecture.

He was a very happy and industrious person who gave a great deal of his life to the study of metaphysics and spirituality. He read voraciously and became extremely knowledgeable in medicine, psychology and religious practices from around the world.

He was also known for his abilities as a psychic and fortune-teller.

Before re-discovering Reiki he'd been running a small business which failed, leaving him deeply demoralised and heavily in debt.

As many people do, when life seems to be letting them down, he sought help and guidance from 'Higher Sources'.

He wanted to know what life was all about. And it was to Mount Kurama that he went to seek his answers, for it was well known in the area as a place of spiritual enlightenment.

Dr Usui's Satori

At that time it was not unusual for people to go on a twenty-one day meditation and fasting retreat on the mountain, and it was known that Dr Usui had a favourite place where he liked to meditate.

It was a beautiful spot near a waterfall and it was whilst actually meditating under the waterfall that he had a moment of enlightenment or 'Satori' as it is known in Japanese.

This is when the full realisation of the meaning of life, and the healing system he called Reiki, became known to him.

From this time on Dr Usui used the Reiki energy on himself and then on his friends and family.

As it worked so well he began using it on the general public and eventually opened up his first clinic in Tokyo.

His fame as a healer began to spread, bringing people from far and wide. These people came not only for healing but also to learn the system for themselves.

This led to the founding of the Reiki movement, which Dr Usui called 'Usui Reiki Ryoho Gakkei' (Usui Healing Method Society).

The Tokyo earthquake

In 1923 a powerful earthquake hit Tokyo causing massive damage to the city, with death and injuries to many thousands of inhabitants.

Dr Usui used his Reiki healing to great effect during this time and such was the success of Reiki his first clinic soon became too small to cope...

So a larger one was built in Nakano outside Tokyo!

Usui's fame began spreading even further now; indeed his name began to be known throughout Japan.

With this fame came invitations to travel to distant cities, which Dr Usui undertook, and it was while on one of these visits to Fukuyama that he had a stroke and died on March 9th 1926.

Now as you can see, the two versions are quite different.

And, wouldn't you just know it, the proponents of each one claims their version to be the original and genuine article.

So, which one would you like to choose? Either or neither may be the truth.

Whilst you're deciding let's give you another issue to consider.

Western Reiki has recently 'discovered', that Reiki still exists in Japan. It hadn't died out in the Second World War as was originally believed.

Inevitably this has led to comparisons between the two styles.

There are differences, of course, bringing about the almost obligatory; 'Ours is better than yours' game being played by both sides.

If this weren't so sad it would be laughable.

Reiki is supposed to enlighten, for God's sake, and we really do mean - for God's sake. This childish nonsense has no place in Reiki and should be firmly set aside.

Reiki is the energy of the Divine. It cares not one jot as to how or where it is brought into the lives of those who have chosen to receive it.

Reiki simply enters and works regardless.

So, just know and understand this...

Reiki as taught and practised in the West WORKS.

Reiki as taught and practised in the East WORKS.

It cannot be any other way.

To say any different is to deny the essence of Reiki itself.

Reiki is the life force energy – the life force energy is ALL THAT IS, for in our universe there is only this ONE energy.

Anyone, therefore, saying their method of receiving Reiki is better than another is implying that All That Is shares their jaundiced view.

How arrogant. How misguided.

Okay, we'll put the soapbox away for now. But before we move on let's just cover a few other concerns.

Dr Usui was not a Christian

Dr Usui was almost certainly not a Christian; he was far more likely to have been a Buddhist.

His knowledge of other religions would probably have included Christianity but there is no record of him being Dean of Doshisha University in Kyoto.

It is known he did travel to western countries and China, but there is no record of him attending Chicago University as either a student or lecturer.

He was not a doctor in the conventional western sense, his Japanese students or disciples referred to him as Usui-Sensei (sensei means teacher).

[We have no problem in continuing to call him doctor though, by the way].

Reiki was not just an oral teaching Dr Usui and Dr Hayashi both produced manuals for their students.

No Grand Master Title

There was no title of Grandmaster created; instead there was a president of the Usui Reiki Ryoho Gakkei. Dr Usui was, quite obviously, the first president and there have been six further presidents: Mr Ushida, Mr Taketomi, Mr Watanabe, Mr Wanami, Mrs Koyama and finally Mr

Kondo who is the present president at the time of writing.

Reiki did not die out in Japan and only become available in the West through Mrs Takata, as some people believe.

The existence of the Usui Reiki Ryoho Gakkei now known as Usui Kai confirms this.

Dr Hayashi was not given the title of Grandmaster (for as we have said this title did not and does not exist) he was a respected disciple of Dr Usui who had been granted teacher status. Dr Hayashi did teach Mrs Takata and did pass on the complete teachings to her.

He obviously did not pass on to her the title of Grandmaster.

Dr Usui did not develop the five principles; he adapted them from those of the Meiji Emperor which were:

The five principles of the Meiji Emperor
Don't get angry today.
Don't worry today.
Be grateful today.
Work hard today.
Be kind to others today.

The Reiki taught by Dr Usui probably consisted of the following five items:

1. The ability to channel the Reiki energy and give Reiki treatments.
2. The attunement symbols and the ability to pass on Reiki to others.
3. The three degrees of Reiki.
4. The five Reiki principles.
5. The necessity to charge for a treatment

Dr Hayashi added the twelve hand positions of Reiki through his observations on healing taking place in his clinic.

Mrs Takata introduced the high fee structure of $10,000 for taking the Reiki Master attunement

Students of Mrs Takata introduced the required waiting times between the classes for the attunements.

A clearer picture?

We hope this is beginning to bring a somewhat clearer picture of Reiki history to those people who may already be involved in the art, and who might have received mixed messages from others.

If you are new to Reiki, please ignore and forgive the political wrangling and just enjoy Reiki for what it is.

Drawing some final conclusions

As you can now see, Traditional Reiki, if there could ever be such a thing, can probably only be the Reiki as taught by Dr Usui.

He taught his students how to use the Reiki energy for healing, both themselves and others, and the three degrees of Reiki (although in Japan they teach six).

The ability to pass the energy on to others through the attunement processes.

The five principles of Reiki, sometimes known as the Reiki Ideals.

And possibly the notion that people have to pay for Reiki treatments.

As far as we are aware at this time, that's it.

That is the entirety of Reiki as originally taught by Dr Usui to over 2000 people.

He almost certainly did not teach crystal grids, psychic surgery, the healing attunement, the Antahkarana, Tibetan Reiki, Karuna Reiki, Seichem, Tera-Mai,

Raku Kei, Sekhem, Advanced Reiki or any of a host of other techniques and trainings now available.

All of these are add-ons and have been introduced by other Reiki Masters who have followed on after.

Most of these additions are quite valid in their own right and can be extremely useful.

Some, like the splitting up of Reiki into many more levels is not.

That, to us, would appear to be just going for the money!

It also has to be taken into account that Dr Usui was a great student of metaphysics and spirituality, and, from what we can make out, very eclectic in nature...

So, the probability is very high he might have gone on to expand Reiki by including these extras himself, had they proved to be useful.

As far as we are concerned, bringing Reiki into your life is and always should be a wonderful experience.

For us it's simply the act of experiencing All That Is more directly. It has nothing to do with religion of any kind. All That Is is not accessible purely through religion.

For us Reiki simply means this:

Personal Communion with All That Is

This is, of course, our interpretation of the word.

You see, in Japan, Reiki is a generic term for healing; which is why the Reiki founded by Dr Usui was called Usui Shiki Ryoho (Usui System of Natural Healing).

Interpreting the word Reiki

In Japanese the Kanji Ideogram Rei apparently can be interpreted as having several meanings, (and we say apparently because we cannot read Japanese ourselves and have to rely on others).

Anyway, the meanings for Rei are - universal, holy, spiritual consciousness.

The kanji for Ki can mean - energy, life force, vital force that animates all living things.

So from this it can be seen that the word Reiki can be translated into – the universal and holy, spiritually conscious, life force energy that energises and animates all living things.

Are there many more apt descriptions of All That Is?

Even if you are someone who can't, at the moment, bring yourself to believe in such an entity, or prefer to use another name.

There we are then, that's the potted history of Reiki.

But don't take any of it too seriously.

Just remember, Reiki was not 'invented' by Dr Usui, it was already there. He merely discovered or, more accurately, re-discovered a method for allowing it more consciously into his life.

Reiki does not, indeed cannot, belong to any one society, country or person.

It belongs to everyone.

To imagine differently would be like believing only members of a certain religion have the right to breathe the air. Reiki, just like air, is everywhere and can be drawn upon by anyone at any time.

So, let's leave these thorny issues there for now and get down to…

The Reiki Attunement

Okay then. First of all we'll introduce you to the symbols as used in Western Usui Reiki.

Now please understand...

These symbols are only like switches; they do not hold the power of Reiki within them. These symbolic switches serve only to focus and concentrate your intention.

Remember – always remember - you are the only power in your universe.

So, practice drawing the following symbols and get to the stage where you can easily do it from memory.

The simplest way is to take just one symbol at a time and keep on copying it out until it fixes in your mind.

Don't try to rush this process, there's no need to hurry.

Trying to cram them all into your head at one sitting will probably end up with you being totally confused.

As you draw each one say its Sacred Name over and over, so as this too lodges in your memory.

When you feel confident in your ability to draw them on paper from memory -

practice drawing them out in front of you, in the air.

There are several ways you can do this.

You can use your fire finger, which is your middle finger – the palm of your hand – your eyes - the tip of your nose – the tip of your tongue – or you can just see each Symbol fully formed in your mind's eye.

Whichever method you choose, and there are no rights or wrongs here, hold the intention that the Symbol is really being drawn out in front of you.

Chapter 15: Meditation And Reiki

Meditating means thinking about something concrete in order to understand the in-depth meaning. In the Western world, meditating means concentrating on a thought, a word, or a situation, discarding any other reflection, in order to reach an altered state of consciousness.

Meditation is an adventure, the greatest adventure that the human mind can reach. Teenagers are usually fascinated with sexuality, money, and material goods, but, over time, they discover that these do not give them full happiness, so they begin to look for it in spirituality. Meditation is not an escape from economic and social problems: it must be synonymous with joy for everyone, not fatigue or boredom.

Meditation makes our being in harmony with the universe. These results can be obtained through numerous techniques, some of the Western origin.

In Eastern tradition, meditation means doing nothing to reach a state of perfect inner peace, to a special state in which the mind is absent and silent. It's a situation in which an indescribable feeling of deep peace and happiness is experienced.

The meditative state is very personal and occurs in each of us in a unique way. Sometimes, it is difficult to attempt a description of what happened. With meditation, we will feel calmer and more aware. We will sleep better, we will get tired less, and our aura will begin to vibrate in a more harmonious way, reflecting spiritual growth. In an easier and different way of relating to our fellow men, we will raise our immune level, causing the body cells to work in a uniform and balanced way. Reiki can be a way to perform deep meditation.

By activating Reiki after the meditations, we will feel a significant difference by finding ourselves closer and in closer contact with the universe and, therefore, with universal energy. Meditation presupposes a series of things that are common to all methods. The first rule for meditation is a relaxed body, without controlling the mind and without concentrating. The eyes must remain closed, as 85 percent of our contact with the outside is done through the eyes. It is better to find a comfortable position than having to change it during the process. The second is to just observe the mind, a thought, as if it were a film in which we are only observers, without interfering, whatever it is. Observe the mind, without any judgment and without criticism.

Meditation is the simple existence without doing anything, without action, without thought, without emotion, and in the absence of criticism and judgment. Slowly, a deep silence will take possession of us. Those are the three main points: relaxation, observation, and lack of criticism.

Tree Meditation

Sit in a comfortable position, breathe slowly and deeply, and close your eyes. Visualize a tree in front of you and feel your energy. Become that tree. Notice that this tree has a long trunk. Notice the branches and leaves. Feel the roots of that tree as it penetrates the ground and the energy of the earth that is emanated in your direction and is enveloping you.

Now, the roots penetrate more deeply until they reach an underground river. It is a stream of translucent and clear waters. The creek bathes its roots, taking away all its fears, anger, limitations, and sadness. A golden light penetrates its roots, bringing a feeling of peace, well-being, and balance.

Now, move your mind toward the tree trunk again and feel that it is expanding upward, passing even further beyond the clouds, reaching the stars. Feel that the energy from which the star is made is the same as that of your body. Feel in communion with the stars, with the universe. Now, a white light emanates from the cosmos. Feel that energy. Return immediately to the trunk. Perceive, in turn, nature, vegetation, other trees, birds, and other small beings.

Become, in turn, fully aware of all life forms, and share with them the experience you have had. Transmit to all beings the energy of love and communion. Divide it. That energy is inexhaustible.

Return slowly toward your body. Move your feet, hands, and legs. Open and close your eyes until you feel that you have entered the body perfectly.

Chapter 16: An Overview

Reiki is a healing practice which originated from Japan. It is based upon the idea that there is a universal source of energy (often referred to as a life source) which supports our body's ability to heal itself and transfer that energy to another. Its practitioners all seek access to this energy, allowing it to flow freely through the bodies and therefore, be able to facilitate healing.

Although it is typically practiced as a natural form of self-care, it can also be offered as a treatment to another. In fact, it is also often used in a variety of health care settings such as hospitals, medical offices, and clinics. This is also mostly used by itself or in conjunction with other conventional medical treatments or even complementary and alternative medicine (CAM) therapies. A few key points to keep in mind are:

Reiki is often used as a means of promoting overall health and well-being. For the most part, most practitioners use it to relieve different disease-related symptoms as well as some of the side effects of certain conventional medical treatments. It helps the body and the mind recover faster while strengthening it as well.

In order for an individual to be able to perform it, a special background is not needed. In fact, training as well as certification for practitioners is not formally regulated. Don't let this deter you from learning it, however!

Currently, there are a number of scientific studies being done in order to learn more about the possible benefits of Reiki, and how it can further help improve a person's health. Its effects on healing certain diseases and conditions are also being studied.

A Brief History:

The word "Reiki" itself will provide you with valuable insight when it comes to the beliefs and theories at work behind it. It is comprised of two Japanese words: "rei" which means universal and "ki" which means life energy. The current practice can be traced back to Mikao Usui's spiritual teachings which were shared during the early 20th century in Japan. These teachings involved both healing and meditative techniques.

One of his students, Chujiro Hayashi, further developed the healing practices while giving less emphasis to the meditative side of Reiki. It was in the 1930's that it was introduced to the Western culture via Hawayo Takata, one of Hayashi's own students.

Types of Reiki Healing:

There are two types of Reiki healing and these are:

Distant – This can be done regardless of time and place, even without the patient being in the same space as the healer. In this process, the healer would likely ask for certain details about the patient. It could be their name and age. Sometimes, healers would also ask for a photograph which would aid them in healing. This particular method is, of course, not as powerful as when directly using the hands on the patients for healing.

Hands On – This can be compared to touch healing wherein the healer's palms are held at least 3 to 5 inches away from the patient's body. In this method, the healer would channel different points on the patient's body. These points are called chakras and it is believed that when one is compromised, the body manifests this in the form of sickness or lethargy. A group healing for this method is known to be most effective and powerful. This means the more healers attending to a patient at the same time, the more concentrated and better it is.

How Reiki Can Benefit You:

Reiki healing can provide you with energy so that you're more capable of dealing with negative forces that might surround you day in and day out. There are numerous people who have also benefited from Reiki's ability to treat common illnesses such as colds, sinusitis as well as sciatica. Sciatica is characterized by leg pain, numbness, or weakness that starts in the low back and travels down the sciatic nerve in the leg causing the pain. It is also effective when it comes to muscle pain and arthritis. Besides these, some people have also claimed that Reiki helped with their diabetes as well as cancer.

Apart from its healing benefits, Reiki can also aid a person when it comes to their mental, emotional, and spiritual health. It is often used as a means of improving relationships such as marriages or even office matters that can significantly affect the productivity of a particular group.

However, it must be noted that a Reiki healer only provides you with energy. Ultimately, it still depends on you to help yourself. So if subconsciously you're not willing to heal then nothing can help. And it is for this reason that healers never promise nor will they guarantee positive results from every session.

What is Reiki Attunement?

This is the process in which an individual becomes a Reiki healer, and their chakras open up. One of the main differences between healing and attunement is that healing provides energy to help heal while an attunement uses the same energy to turn another into a healer.

There is very little formal education when it comes to learning the practice. Typically, your teacher would provide a short lecture on what Reiki is, along with its history and different levels. Afterward, a demonstration and hands on practice is done in order for the person to be able to practice the different hand techniques.

Chapter 17: Reiki: In-Depth Explanation

Reiki does not appeal to a specific type of person. Its benefits do not change based on things like age, demographics, or religion. Reiki works on the spiritual life energy that flows through all of us. You do not have to be religious to practice Reiki, nor do you have to be certified. You can practice Reiki by yourself simply by knowing how.

Now that you know Reiki can help everyone, you may be wondering how exactly it can benefit you. Read on to learn some of the many benefits of this ancient Japanese technique.

#1: Reiki Allows You to Rise to Life's Challenges

When you practice this Japanese healing art long-term, you are better equipped to rise to life's challenges. As healing energy flows through you, you will experience a clarity of mind that will come to you in some of your most trying times. You will find yourself looking at problems in terms of how you can solve them, rather than panicking about what you are going to do next.

#2: Reiki Allows You to Uncover Your Strengths

When you practice Reiki, you are establishing a much deeper spiritual connection to yourself and the flow of your body. You will learn to look deeply at yourself in terms of what you are able to accomplish. You will not foster doubts, but instead will uncover all of your attributes that make you strong enough to excel in the life path of your choosing.

#3: Reiki Can Grant You Inner Peace

As you continue to practice the Japanese practice of Reiki, you will find yourself connecting more deeply with your inner spiritual self than ever before. You will reach a deeper understanding of who you are as a person and come to terms with the person that you are. You may even find insight as to the reasons you think or behave the way that you do. Coming to terms with who you are and why you are the way you are, will give you a newfound confidence in yourself and grant you peace with your inner self.

#4: Reiki Can Alleviate the Symptoms of Chronic Illness

Chronic illness is defined as a long-term illness that lasts for three months or longer, with some of them lasting the patient's lifetime. Chronic illnesses are often accompanied by pain, fatigue, and other symptoms. Reiki has been shown to improve pain management, reduce stress, increase relaxation, and enhance your sense of well-being. Some illnesses benefited by Reiki include:

Chronic pain (back, hip, neck, shoulder, etc.)

Heart disease

Cancer

Irritable bowel syndrome (IBS)

Crohn's disease

HIV/AIDS

Traumatic brain injuries

Developmental delays and disorders like Autism

Chronic fatigue

#5: Reiki Can Help Manage Mental Illness and Stress

Reiki has been shown to significantly improve mental illness for a number of reasons. It calms the mind, allows one to think more clearly, reduces stress, and improves your attitude by helping you think in more a positive way. Some of the mental stresses known to be benefited by Reiki include:

Anxiety disorders

Depression

Mild psychosis

Emotional illness and behavioral disorders

#6: Reiki Allows Positivity to Flow Through Your Entire Life

As you practice Reiki more, you will find that your ability to sense the spiritual energy flowing through your body increases. As you feel this, you can simply imagine that it is a positive force flowing through your body. You will find that the positivity stays with you longer after each session, until it flows into all areas of your life.

#7: Reiki Promotes Personal Growth

Those who practice Reiki understand themselves deeper than they ever would have before. If you choose to, it can allow you to explore the depths of your soul and uncover the things you would like to change about yourself. As you uncover these things, your practice will allow you to change them by giving you time to reflect. You may even set your intent to promote your own personal growth, which you will learn about in Step 3.

Are you ready to get started learning the techniques that will allow you to reap the many benefits of Reiki? Keep reading!

Chapter 18: How Is Healing Expected To Be Obtained From Using This Medication Techniques

Rebalances Chakras
The capacity of Reiki to rebalance the chakras gives creative advantages to another slate. While promoting the self-confidence needed for unbridled speech, chakras that are balanced and spinning merrily improve the link to creative energies. By invigorating and unifying the body, mind, and spirit, all types of creativity can blossom fully. Dancers are able to dance more freely, painters are able to paint more deeply, and authors can write more deeply.
Quiets the Monkey Mind
In the any process , the restless, relentless chatter of the mind can bring a large dent. Reiki can take care of it, calming the constant stream of fear, self-doubt, and other intrusive thoughts of the mind. Once

the mind is quiet, from a powerful and grounded base, you can explore the universe much easier.

Reiki Sensations

As Reiki energies flow throughout the Reiki session between the physician and the recipient, the two bodies may respond or react with specific sensations. These feelings are almost always enjoyable. You may feel heat, warmth, cold, subtlety, stamina, or strength. The fact that you can feel that Reiki flows, whether you give it or receive it, is to verify that the energy is being welcomed.

What Reiki Feels Like

Reiki experience is as distinctive as everyone who receives Reiki. People have recorded common sensations such as feeling heat or coolness, tingling, vibration or noise, itchiness and/or somnolence. During the meeting, some individuals reported "feeling" nothing physical but after the session was over, they noticed beneficial modifications.

Reiki operates like a body regulating the thermostat. As a furnace, that toggles between on and off automatically to control the temperature, Reiki flows slowly or quickly, as needed, to

dispense balancing energies. Reiki sometimes moves erratically, sometimes smoothly, like a pendulum swinging back and forth. Whether you're getting fed up, chills

Using Reiki to Assist with a Career Change
Whether you're fed up, burned out, or just finally gathered the confidence to call it quits at your current job, your cards may have a career change. And if you use Reiki to assist you both target your dream job and set you up for achievement, you have a nice opportunity to play those cards right. While it can be an interesting prospect to change careers, it is also one that can take an avalanche of stress and fear just as rapidly. Leaving your ancient job behind and its safety can begin the engine of stress and fear, which turns into complete gear when you start bombarding your mind with a host of issues:

Should I go for something that I enjoy or make me wealthy? What if this fresh career bored me?

Does anybody even hire?

What kind of training, training, and abilities do I need? Will I create sufficient cash to survive?

What if I fail and end up breaking up, living alone and somewhere on the side of a highway?

Improve This with Letting Go and Letting Higher Energy Flow

For performers, additional blocks may include fear of making a mistake, perfectionism, or otherwise becoming so strongly invested in a project's outcome that they are too paralyzed to even make the first step. Reiki can increase creativity by promoting relaxation by assisting you to let go of the result, the need to adequately perfect, the fear, and other barriers that may hinder the creative process. You are more easily able to link with your intuition when your resistance to letting go and being your true self is relinquished. You can also let something greater shine through than yourself. You can be open to the beautiful instead of attempting to manage your creative output.

Letting Go of the "I"

Reiki's entire scheme is about letting go of the "I".

This was noted out very obviously by Mikao Usui within the precepts:

- Don't be upset.
- Don't be afraid.
- Be thankful.
- Do this conscientiously.
- Show yourself and others kindness

If we only look at the precepts at a superficial level, we won't see that they're leaving the "I" absent, but if we look more deeply into them, we can see that clearly. Let's ask some questions for ourselves and see what the responses are.

Who gets worried? I get worried. Who's getting upset? I'm getting upset.

Who wouldn't be thankful? I'm not thankful.

Who's sympathetic in the manner? I'm sympathetic in my manner.

Who is not diligently practicing? I'm not in the manner of diligent practice.

Reiki Precepts – A Deeper Perspective

Looking deeper into it, we can slowly start to see that this is why the precepts are about leaving the "I." If we remove the "I," then we find that there is no "I" that gets angry or worried. In the way of being grateful, not living diligently, or being compassionate, there is no "I."

It seems, however, that we often try to strengthen the grip on the "I" in many Reiki system doctrines, rather than gradually (and maybe one day completely) letting go of the "I." Looking at an example of other hands-on healing.

When we feel something while doing practical healing on others, we often begin labeling what we feel; for instance, we may feel something and label it heat. We could say to ourselves as quickly as we label it heat; "because I feel the heat, I need to use this symbol now." Or we could say: "because I feel the heat this means my client has a severe problem."

Labeling, separating and judging all come from the "I" —I feel this and so I'm going to do it to my customer. Apart from being "doing" rather than "being," we tighten our grip on the "I" by labeling, distinguishing and judging. So we can also ask some easy questions for ourselves: Who is labeling? Who distinguishes? Who is it that judges? The response to all these questions is "I am."

Been Mindful

In his teaching, Mikao Usui also added methods of mindfulness, such as Joshin Kokyu Ho, or focused on a mantra or symbol. "Awareness needs observation, but it must be free from interpretation and judgment." -Tarthang Tulku These methods of awareness are also there to assist us to let go of the "I" so that we can achieve the ultimate teachings within the Reiki scheme: Just be.

Simply be.

When we're just simply being with our client, we begin to enter a state of unity that can't occur when the "I" is engaged. Because once there's an "I," there's an "I" and "you" and suddenly we're distinct. Being Reiki is the essence of the teachings of Mikao Usui, but to be alone we must let go of the "I." QUESTION: Does letting go of the "I" mean we're losing our distinctive humanity

— say, our beliefs, our lovely singing voice, our chocolate ice cream love? And when we go through our lives, become a bland, nameless, faceless individual with no views?

No; it just implies that we're letting go of attachments to ideas like, "I'm more aged and experienced than you because I've been practicing for 5 years and you've just begun," "My voice is more enjoyable to listen to than yours because I've got an ideal pitch," or "I have a more advanced palate than you because I like chocolate and you like vanilla." While each of these– compare, label, distinguish, judge–may be true to our human minds, they all believe Separateness is a cloud.

And secretly holding on to "I" and "you" – is like attempting to hold on to a cloud, something that is going to come and go temporarily. If instead we practice "free of interpretation and passing judgment" consciousness, if we practice Reiki's system in this way, we can begin to loosen our grip on the "I" and hold on to something that has always been and is with us, our True Self. We can just Be.

Chapter 19: Using Reiki On Yourself

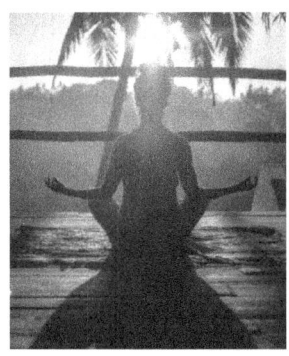

In order to perform Reiki on yourself, you need to lay your hands in the indicated order.

To perform positions that are difficult to reach, for example, on the back, you should put your hands nearby and imagine that 'the hands are in the correct position'. Reiki energy will go to the place you are thinking of. Reiki can instantly pass through either hands laid on, or through the realization that Reiki healing is directed to a specific position.

The time for transferring Reiki energy to the main positions for those who completed the first stage is basically five minutes (60 minutes in total for all stages). It has been experimentally established that this period of time is most effective. However, you can determine the time that is right for you, as it depends on individual abilities.

After you have sent Reiki to all the main positions, put your hands on the sore spots. If you do not have enough time, put your hands on the sore spot immediately after directing energy to the head area. There is no set time period for this. Hands are usually removed after you have a feeling of healing or relief (a feeling of some effect).

Imagine that the treatment is very easy and feel that you can easily perform it anytime, anywhere. You can get some exposure even after healing for as little as five minutes in one position if you are in a hurry. And although to establish complete harmony it is necessary to fulfill all the main positions of Reiki treatment at a time, they are allowed to be performed separately at different times. Performing the treatment daily helps to heal the mind and body, relieve unnecessary stress, and increase your spirituality.

Standard hand positions are used not only to treat patients but also for self-healing. At the same time, in the position on the shoulders, you cannot cross your arms, each palm rests on its side. A phantom arm is used to treat hard to reach areas on the back. A phantom stands out from the physical arm in that we simply 'know' that our arm lies on the right part of the body. Reiki flow will be felt both in the position of the phantom arm and out of the palm of the physical arm, the phantom of which is used for treatment. Do not forget to "take" the phantom of your hand - just pulling it into the physical hand with intent.

Be sure to ground yourself at the end of self-healing. For those who are still struggling to bend to their feet, you can use the front lower leg area below the knee to ground, just understanding what needs to be done.

Hand Positions for Healing

Standard hand positions:

- Two palms on the parietal bones, not closing the median line and Sahasrara
- Two palms on the temporal bones (covering the ears)
- Two palms on the occipital bone (support the back of the head)
- The left hand on the back of the head opposite Ajna (6th chakra) (or center of the forehead), the right on the front of the head
- Left behind the neck. Right in front of the neck. (Vishuddha (5th chakra), middle of the neck)
- Hands on shoulders (this is a very wobbly position for filling the whole body with Reiki energy)
- Hands in the area of Anahata (4th chakra)
- Hands in the area of Manipura (3rd chakra)
- Hands in the area of Swadhisthana (2nd chakra)

- Hands in the area of Muladhara (1st chakra) (treatment with the touch of a 'phantom' hand or alternating exposure with the right hand through the right and left knee to the left hand on the sacrum is possible)

You can move your hands all over your body. Zones with an energy imbalance will either absorb a lot of power, feel cold, or resist. The healed area is filled with light and warmth and will itself bring you Reiki.

Additional hand positions:

- Hands in the area of the lungs from 2 sides of the spine from the back
- Hands in the area of the kidneys from 2 sides of the spine from the back
- Hands in the area of the pelvic bones from 2 sides of the sacrum from the back
- Hands in the apex of the lungs, under the collarbone from 2 sides of the sternum
- Hands in the area of the liver and pancreas in the diaphragm from 2 sides on the front surface
- Hands in the abdomen from 2 sides of the navel

- Be sure to ground the patient holding his hands on the back of the ankle joints

Schedule of treatment sessions

- Immediately after tuning in to energy level 1, it is imperative to treat yourself for 21 days
- Daily conducting a full Reiki session for yourself will provide you with release from emotional stress, inner peace, endurance, sense of security, joy of life, creative disclosure, detection of hidden abilities, increased sensitivity, development of intuition, neutral, understanding attitude towards people, reduction or disappearance of pain and illness, holistic personality development
- If you are conducting Reiki sessions to another person, then conducting 4-6 full sessions first is effective. After that, you can continue 1-2 times a week
- If the symptoms are acute, treat the attention-grabbing body part for as long as possible, several times a day. If symptoms spread to the whole body (or if the disease is chronic), then a full session is helpful!

- If you have to treat burns, injuries, or infectious skin diseases, then keep your hands at a distance of 1-2 palms from the affected area

How to conduct a Reiki session

In order to call Reiki, it is enough to fold your hands in Gassho (prayer gesture) and repeat this three times (out loud or to yourself): "Reiki! Reiki! Reiki! "- so that the energy hears you and comes to your call.

However, in order to immediately teach the beginner the right attitude towards the Forces that we call upon, Reiki Masters instruct their students to always address Reiki and its Guides personally and consciously.

To do this, various Masters offer their students different options for accessing Reiki energy. However, it is important to remember that not a mechanical repetition of memorized formulations, but sincerity, love, deep respect, and openness of the heart are the key to your success in working with any divine entities, including the Reiki energy.

Beginning of a Reiki session:

Open your palms to increase their sensitivity, fold your hands in Gassho (prayer gesture), respectfully invoke and greet Reiki's energy with these words:

"Here and now I invoke the Divine energy of Reiki, the thin conductors of Reiki, the teachers of Reiki!"

Listen to the sensations in your palms and feel how the energy of Reiki has responded to your call and flowed from your hands.

In this case, additional warmth will appear in the hands, a feeling of slight tingling, a feeling of a special density of space between the hands or something else. These subtle sensations usually appear in all Reiki guides immediately after any invocation and are an indication that Reiki has come to you. If you are just starting your Reiki practice or you mumbled the call mechanically and did not feel any changes in the space between your palms, just repeat the call with concentrated attention. Listen to yourself, and subtle sensations will certainly appear!

Then formulate your intention or wish of your client.

If you are doing a Reiki healing session, your intention might be:

"Here and now I ask You, the divine energy of Reiki, I ask you ... (list your personal Guides) and you, Teachers and Guides of Reiki: heal and harmonize all (my) bodies and shells (or here is the name of your patient), on at all levels and in all spaces!"

"Here and now I ask You, Divine Reiki, harmonize my emotional state, calm my thoughts and feelings. Give me a healthy sleep!"

"Oh Reiki! Heal me from this excruciating headache!"

Reiki Session Itself

Start a Reiki session with your hands on yourself.

Now that you have invoked the energy of Reiki and its Guides, and have formulated your request, you can put your hands on your body, proceeding directly to the Reiki session.

You can conduct a session intuitively (moving your hands, guided by your inner sensations) or make a full session in all positions, as described in the manual. The single rule for all cases is this: stay in one position until you feel that your hands 'want to move on.' This will be a signal that this position has already been sufficiently developed and filled with Reiki. If at first it is difficult for you to track such subtle sensations or you doubt yourself, then you can work in each position from 3 to 5 minutes. Usually, this time is enough to fully saturate the energy of each zone of the body.

When the problem you are working with is local, for example, if your head or back hurts, you can do a short local Reiki session in this area. Such a session can last 15 to 20 minutes, after which, acute pain usually disappears or decreases. Chronic diseases require a longer, systematic, and full-fledged healing, which will require changes in your worldview and lifestyle.

But remember that for Reiki, as well as for God, there is nothing impossible.

When you feel that this Reiki session is coming to an end, or when you have successfully completed all the positions, know that your work is completed and you can thank Reiki.

Before the end of the session, you can 'smooth out' your patient's biofield with several light hand passes from head to toe, thus distributing the transferred energy. Although, this is optional, since Reiki is reasonable, and she herself will go to where her presence will be most needed.

Clasping your hands on your chest again in a prayer gesture, thank the energy of Reiki and all those divine beings that you called before the start of the session with these words:

"I thank you, Reiki energy, I thank you (list your personal Guides), I thank you, Reiki Teachers and Guides for a successful self-healing session (or something else that you asked for).

Ending the Reiki Session

After the Reiki session is completed, especially if you did the Reiki contact session to someone else, you need to clean your hands and all your bio-field of energies that are alien to you. And also, to balance the descending and ascending energy flows. For this:

Wash your palms three times with cool water, visualizing how water penetrates into your hands, taking with you all your client's energy that is alien to you.

If there is no water nearby, you can use the fire, imagining how it burns all the negative that remains in the biofield of your hands. Or the earth, laying hands on it and visualizing how Mother Earth cleans you. As a last resort, you can simply imagine any of the proposed cleaning methods on the mental plane, and it will also cleanse you. Such a procedure usually lasts no more than 1-2 minutes, until the characteristic sensation of 'purity and lightness' in your palms.

After that, proceed to balancing the downward and upward flows.

Having risen or sat with a straight back, imagine how a downward flow of energy - a stream of Cosmos energy - descends from above at infinity above into your 7th chakra. It runs along your spine through your entire body and, leaving the 1st chakra, goes to the very center of the Earth. Towards it rises the upward flow - the flow of energy of the Earth. And, having passed the return path, this stream leaves your crown and rises upward to infinity. Feel yourself a small bead hanging on these streams, and give them one minute to harmonize the speed of their flow through you.

Balance both flows in your subtle body and ground yourself.

Then ask Reiki energy to completely cleanse you of everything negative and accept Reiki souls.

Imagine how a huge waterfall of pure Reiki energy or a powerful stream of its light washes your entire body, all your subtle bodies and shells. He carries with him down - to the center of the Earth - everything that pollutes you. Feel how all your subtle bodies are cleansed and filled with divine energy. How does the state of causeless joy, peace, and bliss come to you?

This way you complete the entire three-stage process of energy purification.

Chapter 20: The Origin And History Of Reiki

People are always working so hard to explain how something began. Where did it come from? Who started it? How was it discovered? The answers are always so different from culture to culture, throughout the course of history, and yet in so many ways, the source is the same. How Reiki was invented comes from one region of origin, that was brought to the light of one man's mind from another origin. Prior to that, there were plenty of other origins of the same principles, with too many different versions to describe it. When you consider the history of the human race, you can see that there are always more than just a few answers to any question, and oddly that many discoveries have occurred simultaneously, and without knowledge, in more than one corner of the world.

The Universal life-force energy that we refer to in Reiki is something that always has been and always will be. The man who created the practice of Reiki and gave it that name, was only one of many who formed a rational explanation for what it is and how to work with it for manifesting healing and transformation. The life-force energy we refer to in this book as Reiki was always a part of our lives and our experience and has seen many different titles, forms and functions.

As you become more familiar with the healing art of Reiki, you can begin to uncover some of the ancient mysteries of how it became known to us today through these terms and methods, as well as search for other practices that involve and include similar theories of working with the healing power of this Universal life-force.

Reiki and the Buddhist Tradition

Buddhism is one of the most notable and recognized religious practices in the world today, boasting several million followers. Buddha was named to be the "Godfather of Holiness" and began the teachings of honoring the light of being, existing in oneness with the Universe and balancing the internal and infinite light of the self. He is known for what we have termed 'enlightenment' and showed by life example, practice and through sacred writings, the elements of what leads one down the path of spiritual awakening and wholeness.

Much of what can be understood about the teachings of Buddha, lead to the concept of light and energy as the essence of the soul matter of all beings, and as we honor that love and light, we have the powerful energy of creation, collective consciousness, and Universal love.

In the Veda, the ancient, sacred texts of the Hindu beliefs, there were several different points made about our energy. The texts themselves are said to have been written with some influence from Buddha who was notorious for his spiritual quest to answer the questions about our inner light as souls. His perception of this "life force" was something that he aimed to teach through his own understanding, but did not teach it through any kind of established structure, or technique.

The reality of these energy centers, or vortexes, as we have learned were termed chakras, were literally buried within the texts and beliefs of the rest of the Hindu religions and were not fully practiced, preached, or presented until much later, as various forms of yoga began to evolve as a result of these texts, and with the creation of Reiki by a Buddhist monk of Japanese origin.

The concept of these "life-force energies" and inner light were concealed within the religions of the Indic culture and did not spread to the West until the mis 20th century.

Japanese Origins

Hundreds of years beyond Buddha in the early 20th century, Mikao Usui was living his life as a Buddhist Monk. It was common for Usui to undergo long periods of meditation, sometimes lasting for days and even weeks, with no food and only water and prayer to sustain him. It was during one of these particularly long fasts that Usui awakened to the journey of enlightenment that would influence the manifestation of Reiki.

According to the tale of Usui, he was wandering in the mountains during his fast that had lasted for 21 days. Usui had originally become a monk, as the story goes, in order to ask the questions about what the Buddha had learned and begun to teach about the miracle of healing that was seen in the religions of Christianity, as well as Buddhism. He was determined to find answers about our energy, where it comes from, and what we can do to understand it.

In the last days of his meditation on the mountainside, looking for the mysteries of our life-force, he had an epiphany, as if struck in his forehead (third eye) by lightening. He had sudden awareness and had the answer to his query. He saw the future Reiki symbols flash before him as if drawn by electric light and readied himself to hurry back to the monastery and discover more about his epiphany and moment of enlightenment.

As the tale continues, he is alleged to have stubbed his toe in his hurried state down the mountainside where he stopped to cup his hands around his foot and stop the bleeding. He apparently channeled the healing life force energy and was able to relieve the pain in his toe and carry forward on his quest back home to reveal his secrets discovered.

No one knows for sure if this is the real tale, and the original stories have been passed down over the last many decades from master to student as part of the ritual of teaching Reiki and giving attunements.

Usui then dedicated the remainder of his life to teaching his discovery and helping to heal others through his understanding of how to become a channel of this life force energy. What began as a sacred understanding of the Buddha's teachings became one man's quest to modify the reality of these concepts and bring them to his work with techniques and tools that could be used to create powerful change in the mind, body and spirit.

Usui was able to help his students understand how to use Reiki as a tool to heal themselves and work on healing others, but he never attuned any other masters except for his successor, Chijiro Hayashi, who worked with Usui until his death.

Reiki's Western Introduction

In the time before the second World War, Hawayo Takata was living a life of pain and misery in Hawaii. Originally from Japan, she was there because of her marriage, and had suffered some very serious and unfortunate losses in her family leading to a life of nervous exhaustion, sickness, disease and several recurring tumors that had to be surgically operated on.

According to her story, as she was about to be wheeled into yet another surgery, she began to hear a voice in her mind that told her not to have the surgery and that it wouldn't be necessary. As a result, she chose to avoid the procedure altogether and found herself guided back to her home in Japan where she discovered Dr. Usui's Reiki clinic for healing.

She accepted the healing services of Master Hayashi and his students and stayed within the clinic for several months. She completely healed from her long list of physical conditions, tumors, disease and emotional issues. This major turn around caused her to changer he life, stay in Japan, and become attuned to Reiki as a practitioner with the lessons from Master Hayashi who was then running the clinic after Usui's death in 1926. Takata eventually returned to Hawaii and founded her own Reiki practice.

She became the next Master, following Hayashi. At that time in the history of Reiki, there were only a handful of Masters and so many students. Takata's granddaughter who was a doctor of medicine, studied to become a Master under her grandmother and the two of them began to teach mastery to anyone willing to learn and teach Reiki to others.

Reiki was not seen outside of Japan, or Takata's Hawaiian practice, until much later, as more Masters in the West began to attune more and more students over the past 5 decades.

From Master to Student

Reiki is passed down through attunement and a specific training module that shows the student clear knowledge and pathways of healing various conditions and ailments. As the practice of Reiki has spread, modern teachings have changed and loosened from the original lectures and daily study of the students under Usui, who required a rigorous schedule for regular prayer, meditation, ritual and instruction.

In today's Western practices, you can learn Reiki and receive attunement in a weekend workshop if you want, or you can have a more in depth, longer term apprenticeship with the right Master for your tutelage. Even with the advent of modern practices and different teaching styles from the original format, the essence and principles of Reiki have not changed. Reiki can't change; it always is, and always will be, Universal life-force energy. Once you are attuned to Reiki, it will never leave you.

The history of Reiki is ancient. The name given to this essential energy by Usui may only be a little over 100 years old, but the principles, concepts and journey of understanding this life-force energy is much older. Origins are often never true beginnings. Reiki itself is as old as time and we can thank many spiritual adventurers for bringing more of this truth into the light over the past several centuries and into our modern world.

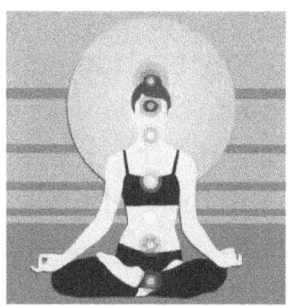

Chapter 21: Origins And History Of Reiki

Reiki is not that old, at least not in comparison to its origins. The history of Reiki is a beautiful and rich weave that dates back to ancient spirituality and sacred religious writings that described the source of our personal power and how we become enlightened. Many people have perceived Reiki as being something that existed in ancient times, farther back than we can truly perceive. Reiki is only about 100 years old, but the discovery of it and the creation of the practice a century ago came from thousands of years prior, and maybe even more than that.

Before I give you all of the Japanese histories of how Reiki was created and evolved into what it has become today, I must first take you back to another land and another time. When you were born, did you know you were here? Most people have no concept of their origin. When we are infants born new into this world we must learn everything from the start, as if we had never been here before.

In Buddhist belief, reincarnation is something that is believed in and described, as well as the description of what our life-force is and why it lies dormant within all of us at the time of our birth. There are a lot of people on Earth and each has a unique energy and life-force that they were born with for a certain purpose, possibly carrying over from a previous existence, but you don't have to believe in reincarnation to practice Reiki. The Buddha was known for his teachings about enlightenment and the concept of awakening to your true purpose through Universal consciousness. But where did these ideas come from?

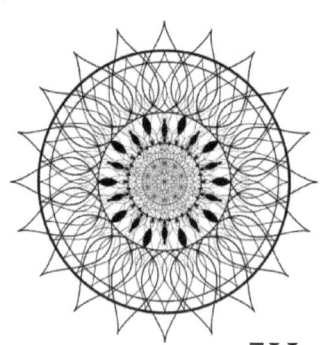

In India, where Buddha lived and taught, philosophies of spirituality and awakening were being written and there were significant similarities in the discoveries of what Buddha had written and what the Upanishad and Vedas of the Hindu religions were stating about our individual spark and the seed of creation. In fact, The Vedas are much older than the teachings of Buddha and it is possible that he was building upon already existing Hindu religious philosophies about what we are and why we are here.

Conclusion

Reiki has a power of healing you which is why it is important to practice it daily as a routine of your life. Just like you have food every day, consider to make Reiki a part of your life as well. Make sure to try it once and if you feel that you cannot live without it then continue it. There are people who have tried and never able to forget it because it actually brings peace to their body and mind. When you are facing any trouble, do not panic instead try to find solutions and there is no better solution then Reiki for you.

This Book is a great guide for you to understand the levels of Reiki as well as the benefits of it. Some people keep on searching for true peace all their life and if you have come across such thing then there is nothing better than getting it instantly and to try it. Learn to take risks in life and see how amazing it turns out to be. You will feel a complete rejuvenation of your soul and body once you get a hold of Reiki and the practice of it. Get in touch with a professional to learn the actual techniques of it and practice them at home.

There will be no hate or anger in you after Reiki is applied on you. You will find solutions for your problems and will want to sort them out as soon as possible. New approaches will take birth from your personality which will amaze you and the people around you for sure. You will see how you quickly you will be able to learn Reiki and apply it on your daily life. There are many hidden benefits of Reiki which you will experience when you are doing it. once you achieve the level of mastery, then you will not be able to leave it even for a day because of the ease it will give you in the most stressful era of all times until now. Do not wait and get started now so that you spend your life happier and enjoy it the most of it.

www.ingramcontent.com/pod-product-compliance
Lightning Source LLC
Chambersburg PA
CBHW052204090526
44583CB00015BA/1330